Intermittent Fasting for Beginners

Simple and Easy-to-Follow Weight Loss Guide on How to Lose Weight Faster, Feel Better and Live a Healthy Lifestyle

Jason Brad Stephens

© **Copyright 2019 by Jason Brad Stephens - All Rights Reserved.**

The contents of this book may not be reproduced, duplicated or transmitted without direct written permission from the author.

Under no circumstances will any legal responsibility or blame be held against the publisher for any reparation, damages, or monetary loss due to the information herein, either directly or indirectly.

Legal Notice:

This book is copyright protected. This is only for personal use. You cannot amend, distribute, sell, use, quote or paraphrase any part or the content within this book without the consent of the author.

Disclaimer Notice:

Please note the information contained within this document is for educational and entertainment purposes only. Every attempt has been made to provide accurate, up to date and reliable complete information. No warranties of any kind are expressed or implied. Readers acknowledge that the author is not engaging in the rendering of legal, financial, medical or professional advice. The content of this book has been derived from various sources. Please consult a licensed professional before attempting any techniques outlined in this book.

By reading this document, the reader agrees that under no circumstances are is the author responsible for any losses, direct or indirect, which are incurred as a result of the use of information contained within this document, including, but not limited to, —errors, omissions, or inaccuracies.

Table of Contents

Introduction

Chapter 1: Getting Started with Intermittent Fasting

Chapter 2: Dealing with Overweight Dilemma

Chapter 3: The Problem with our Diet

Chapter 4: Intermittent Fasting: An Overview on How to Lose Weight Faster

Chapter 5: Intermittent Fasting: Best Foods to Eat

Chapter 6: Intermittent Fasting: Best Time to Eat in a Day

Chapter 7: Picking the Right Meal Plan

Chapter 8: The One Meal a Day approach

Chapter 9: Healthy Recipes

Chapter 10: Mistakes to Avoid and Who Should Not Fast

Chapter 11: When You Are Not Seeing

Results

Chapter 12: Living the Healthy, Guilt-Free Lifestyle

Bonus Chapter: Benefits with Ketogenic Diet

Conclusion

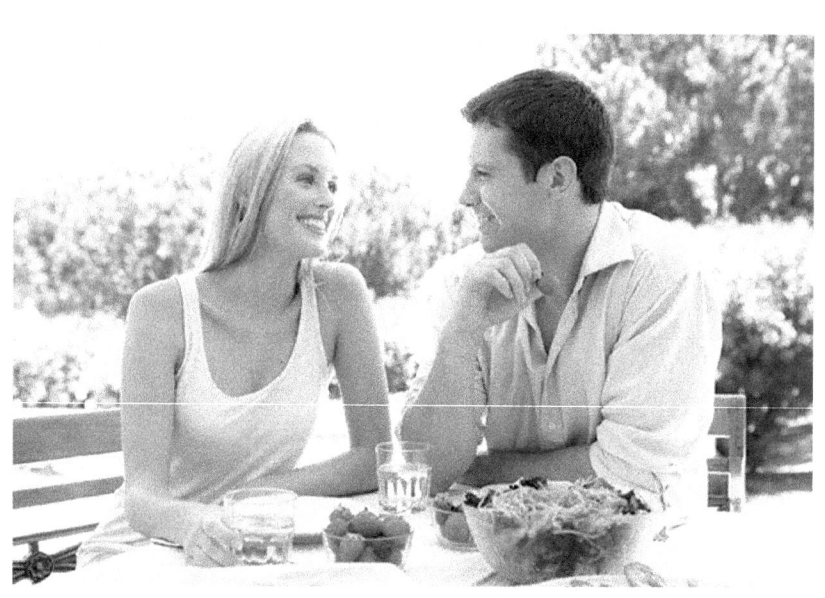

Introduction:

According to a study that was conducted by the World Health Organization, it was revealed that in 2016, more than 1.9 billion adults, aged above 18 years from across the globe, were overweight. 39% of adults aged above 18 years were overweight and 13% were obese in 2016. Worse still, 41 million children aged below 5 years were either overweight, or obese.

Nonetheless, all hope is not lost, as the problem of obesity is preventable. Today, we are experiencing a fitness revolution in many parts of the world as people are becoming more aware of the dangers that a sedentary lifestyle poses to human health. People are taking up fitness, yoga, rhumba, and even Zumba classes, hoping to shed a couple of kilos and to tone their bodies. However, one important point that many people fail to understand is that weight loss is a three-part process that involves fitness and physical activity, a positive mindset and, most importantly, diet. Your diet, both the quality and quantity, is very important in your weight loss program. It will determine how fast you lose weight, and if you will regain the weight that you have lost.

While there are many factors that cause obesity, it is scientifically proven that obesity is hormonal, and not a result of calorie imbalance or excessive consumption of calories. When we eat, the food is broken down and converted into glucose, which is a source of energy for the body. Insulin is a hormone that is involved in the absorption of glucose, and the storage of excess glucose as fats. Hence, it causes cells in the body to absorb this glucose for energy. However, when we eat excessively, the insulin in the bloodstream increases, signaling the body to store most of this glucose as fat, contributing to obesity.

Having seen that insulin is responsible for most cases of obesity, the natural solution is to find ways that will reduce the amount of insulin in the bloodstream. Two of the most common ways of reducing insulin levels in the bloodstream are: the ketogenic diet, and the intermittent fasting diet.

Intermittent fasting is characterized by distinct periods of eating and fasting. It is an important tool that involves calorie restriction, alternating between regular feeding days and fasting days, or limiting the number of hours that you get to eat within the day. There are different methods of intermittent fasting, each with its own distinct characteristics and dietary requirements. They include: the popular 16/8 (which has different variants), the eat-stop-eat method, the 5:2 method, the 4:3 method, and meal skipping, amongst others.

According to Jimmy Moore, fasting is not just any other "F-word". It is a method that dates back to the times of the ancient Greeks and the Egyptians that has proven itself time and time again. Many people who hear the word "fasting" believe that it is synonymous with starvation. However, this book will take you through the fundamental differences between these two concepts and explain to you just why intermittent fasting could be the saving grace of all humanity.

One of the main reasons why intermittent fasting has quickly risen in popularity is that it not only allows you to lose weight, but also improves your health and general well-being. The diet has been associated with increased metabolism, reduced insulin resistance, reduced inflammation, retarded growth of cancer cells, a reduced risk of developing heart diseases, anti-aging and, of course, weight loss.

The diet calls for highly nutritious foods and recipes which should contain both the macro and micronutrients. The meals should be high in proteins, healthy fats, and oils, but low in carbohydrates. This allows the body to remain in a state of ketosis where it burns down the fat reserves for energy, instead of relying on glucose from carbohydrates. Proteins are particularly important, as they nourish the muscles and the body's organs, while creating a feeling of satiation. This reduces hunger pangs and cravings. Some of the foods that are strictly forbidden in this diet include: white foods, fatty cuts of beef and pork, carbonated drinks, and all foods that are rich in starches and simple sugars.

It is arguable that the most important aspect of the intermittent fasting diet is developing the discipline and willpower to stick to the diet, despite the cravings and hunger pangs that people experience. This is because hunger is a powerful feeling that can demotivate and disorient you.

Many people cite that the most difficult aspect of the diet is not the hunger that you experience, but instead is the sheer determination that it will take for you to overcome the conventional three-meals-a-day habit.

The main reason why the intermittent fasting diet fails is because people give in to their bodily urges and social demands in relation to food. Inconsistency, and the inability to follow through with your caloric restrictions, will set you up for failure.

Due to the extreme nature of the intermittent fasting diet, it is not recommended for all people. If you are known to have a history of an eating disorder, or are underweight, this diet may not be for you. Pregnant and lactating women too should avoid this diet. All women should carefully approach this diet as there are instances where it interferes with the natural menstrual cycle. People who suffer from type 2 diabetes, or any other medical conditions, should also approach the diet with caution. Generally, it is highly recommended that you seek the advice of a medical practitioner before starting the diet.

In this book, we aim to provide conclusive knowledge of the intermittent fasting diet, while clarifying some of the myths and misconceptions that are often related to this topic. As a bonus, we will also analyze the ketogenic diet, clearly highlighting why the two diets are the most effective in weight loss.

Chapter 1: Getting Started with Intermittent Fasting

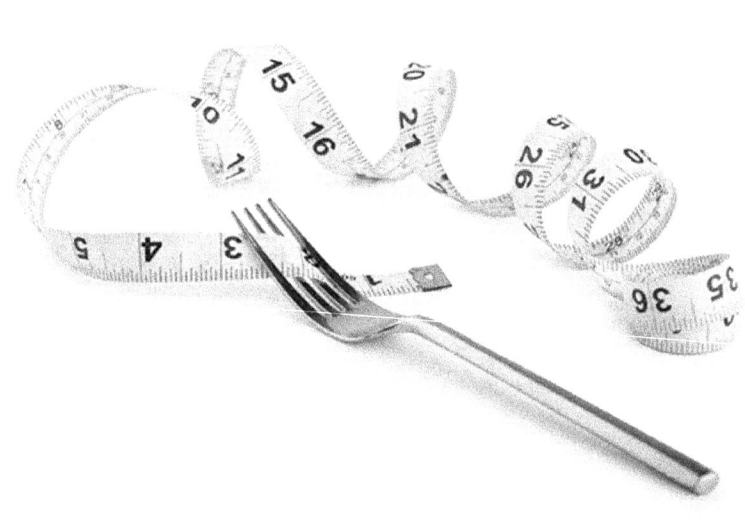

Chapter 1: Getting Started with Intermittent Fasting

1.1 Fasting: Definition and a Brief History

Many people use the word fasting interchangeably with the word starvation. People who use a fasting diet to lose weight will claim, jokingly, that they are starving themselves to lose weight. In such a situation, the correct terminology is fasting, and not starving.

Fasting is fundamentally different from starvation in one way: the ability to exercise control. Starvation refers to the involuntary abstention from eating. Starving people have no idea where, or when, they will have their next meal. Their failure to eat is neither deliberate, nor controlled. Fasting is the *voluntary* abstention from eating. When fasting, food is readily available, but you deliberately choose not to eat it. It is usually done for spiritual, health, and other reasons.

The concept of fasting dates to the days of the ancient Greeks when devotees believed that the practice brought about physical and spiritual renewal.

Fasting has also played a major role in some religions, where it is believed to be a sign of penitence and self-control. In Islam, Muslims fast during the holy month of Ramadhan. The Roman Catholics observe the 40-day fast during the Lenten season. In Judaism, the Day of Atonement is marked as an annual fast day.

Modified fasting, also known as intermittent fasting, is a dietary pattern that involves cycles of eating and fasting. There are different methods of going about intermittent fasting. They include: the 16/8 method, the eat-stop-eat method, the 5:2 diet, and the 4:3 diet. However, the underlying principle is that all these methods split either the day or the week into distinct periods of eating and fasting.

Limiting food intake to the middle of the day, which is a form of intermittent fasting, decreases body weight and fat, glucose and insulin levels, insulin resistance, and inflammation. This leads to mild calorie restriction without necessarily counting calories. Consistency in intermittent fasting is therefore very important for one to lose weight. It is more of a lifestyle than it is a short-term diet.

While intermittent fasting is a conscious effort to skip meals, or to exclusively eat at certain times of the day, regular fasting involves abstaining from food for longer durations of time, mostly days.

While fasting, the calorie intake is usually zero. The body shifts to a state of ketosis where any stored body fat is burned to produce ketones for energy. Fasting may seem to be the quicker way to lose excess weight. It can be detrimental in the long run because it depletes all the glycogen stored in the liver, and the body could begin breaking down its own muscles and organs for energy.

1.2 Benefits of Intermittent Fasting

In the past, humans engaged in food-seeking which would last anywhere from a couple of hours to a few days. The mechanisms that allowed humans to survive such periods of fasting are believed to have numerous benefits, which have been negated by the present-day sedentary lifestyle characterized by continuous and abundant food supply.

Based on a scientific study by, intermittent fasting could lead to:

- An extended lifespan. Intermittent fasting diets are believed to alter the mitochondrial networks inside the energy producing cells, increasing lifespan and promoting good health.
- Protection from obesity, cardiovascular disease, diabetes, and hypertension. During intermittent fasting, the insulin levels in the blood drop significantly, facilitating fat burning. The drop in insulin consequently leads to a drop in blood sugar levels, which decreases the risk of type 2 diabetes. A drop in insulin levels also leads to an increase in the breakdown of body fat, facilitating the use of fat as an energy source. This

greatly reduces the cholesterol levels in the body, and cases of obesity and cardiovascular diseases.

- Improvement in insulin sensitivity. As a result of the decreased insulin levels in the bloodstream, the cells become more sensitive to any insulin released into the bloodstream. As such, it does not accumulate within the blood.
- Retarded growth of tumors. Periodic fasting leads to a decrease in the growth of cancerous tumors and increased sensitivity to chemotherapy. When cancerous cells are exposed to environments that contain lower glucose levels, proliferation and cell death quickly follow. This is a process known as cell starvation.
- Reduced inflammation. Inflammation is a common symptom of all chronic diseases that we face today. It is known to occur whenever the body is trying to heal itself. However, whenever inflammation

occurs for too long, it is associated with some negative effects.

- An intermittent fasting diet involves increased consumption of foods that are rich in fats and oils. These high fats and oils decrease the production of Leukotriene B4 (LTB4) which is involved in various cellular processes that are related to inflammation.
- Enhanced brain functionality. In addition, through intermittent fasting, we have a significant decrease in inflammatory markers such as cytokines and C-reactive protein.
- Improved brain functionality and cognitive functions. Intermittent fasting, just like exercising, leads to the production of a protein called brain-derived neurotrophic factor (BDNF) within the nerve cells. This protein is especially important in learning, memory, and in the production of new nerve cells in the hippocampus.

Other benefits of intermittent fasting include: improving the circulation of cholesterol and triglycerides, resistance to ischemic injury, improved survival from myocardial ischemia, efficient metabolism, and reduced oxidative stress. Hence, we see that intermittent fasting is an effective and convenient lifestyle habit that will make your life simpler, while also improving your health.

1.3 Types of Intermittent Fasting

Intermittent fasting has grown in popularity as one of the recommended ways to lose weight while improving your health and general well-being. Some of the popular methods are:

1. The 16/8 method:

    This is believed to be the most popular method, owing to its sustainability and ease of application. It involves restricting the consumption of foods and calorie-containing beverages to eight hours per day and abstaining from food for the remaining 16 hours. For example, one may decide to eat food between noon and 8 PM only.

During the 8-hour eating period, one should focus on eating healthy meals and drinking calorie-free drinks such as water and unsweetened teas and coffee.

However, the windows may vary from one person to the next, with some people preferring to eat within a 6 hour window (18/6), and others preferring to eat over a 4 hour window (20/4). Nonetheless, the method is easy to follow and provides results with minimal effort.

2. Eat-stop-eat:

This is a form of intermittent fasting that was put together by Brad Pilon. It involves fasting for 24-hour periods either once or twice a week. On the other five or six days, one should concentrate on eating responsibly while keeping the overall calorie intake with the desired range.

The fast can begin either at breakfast, lunch, or dinner, as long as an individual fasts for 24 consecutive hours. During your fasting days, you must make sure to take in as few calories as possible. It is recommended that you should only drink plain or sparkling water, unsweetened tea or coffee, and diet soda. It is important to note that you should break your fast with a regularly sized meal. Avoid compensating for the fast by feasting on a large meal.

3. The 5:2 diet:

    It is also known as the fast diet and is currently the most popular intermittent fasting diet. The diet involves 5 normal eating days and 2 days in which calorie intake is restricted to 500-600 calories per day, or to 25% of your daily calorie intake.

    The choice of eating and fasting days is entirely at your discretion, as long as there is a non-fasting day between any two consecutive fasting days. During normal eating days, you should stick to healthy foods and calorie-free drinks, or else you will not lose any weight at all.

This diet is easier to stick to, as opposed to traditional calorie-restricted diets.

4. The 4:3 diet:

    Also known as the alternate day fasting, this involves a normal eating day followed by a fasting day. This method, though effective for weight loss, is an extreme form of intermittent fasting and is not suitable for beginners or people with different health conditions. In addition, it may be difficult to maintain this kind of diet long-term.

    On the normal days, you are advised to eat as much you want. On the fasting days, you are advised to eat a 400-calorie meal and a 100-calorie snack, to drink lots of water, tea and coffee, and to chew sugarless gum. However, some people recommend completely avoiding solid foods on fasting days.

5. Meal Skipping

This is a method that is especially common among beginners. It involves skipping specific meals of the day depending on your level of hunger or time constraints. In addition, the meals consumed must be healthy to ensure the success of the diet.

The diet plan is especially successful when you keep track and respond moderately to your hunger needs. This implies that you only eat food when you are hungry and otherwise avoid any food.

6. The Warrior Diet

This is an extreme form of intermittent fasting diet that was developed in 2001 by Ori Hofmekler. The diet involves eating small portions of raw fruits and vegetables during a 20-hour fasting period and eating one large meal at night during a 4-hour eating period. It can therefore be described as a cycle of fasting and overeating.

During the 20-hour fasting period, you should consume small amounts of dairy products, hard-boiled eggs, raw fruits and vegetables, and calorie-free fluids. On the other hand, during the 4-hour eating period, you should consume plenty of fruits, vegetables, proteins, and healthy fats. Carbohydrates should also be consumed, though in fewer quantities. The diet is based on the fact that humans are nocturnal eaters and absorb nutrients at night in line with the circadian rhythms. It is mainly used by individuals who have tried other intermittent fasting diets. Beginners should therefore proceed with caution.

Your Quick Start Action Step:

Now it is your turn! Try either one of the above methods of intermittent fasting and record the results from each of the methods, identifying the one that works best for you.

It is important to note that before trying any intermittent diet, you should consult your medical practitioner for the go-ahead.

Inasmuch as intermittent fasting diets are known to be beneficial in the control and management of type-2 diabetes, patients should first consult the advice of a medical practitioner.

Chapter 2: Dealing with the Overweight Dilemma

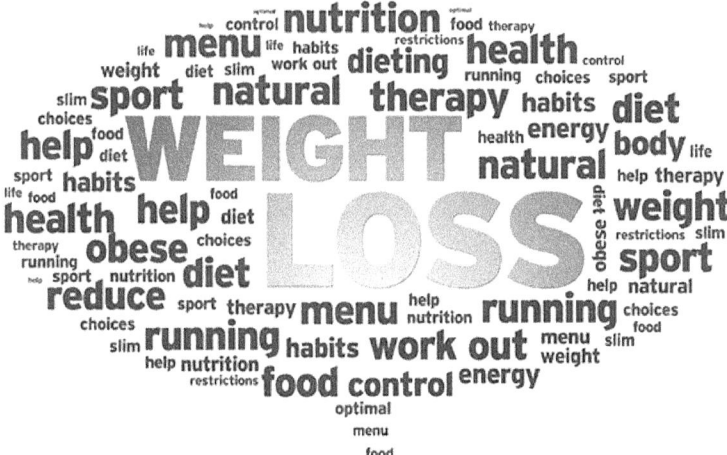

Chapter 2: Dealing with the Overweight Dilemma

2.1 Obesity: Current Issues

Obesity refers to a condition or disorder in which excessive body fat accumulates to the extent in which it may have adverse effects on the general health of an individual. Doctors suggest that anyone with a Body Mass Index (BMI) of between 25 and 29.9 is overweight, while anyone with a BMI above 30 is obese.

According to the newly released Global Nutrition Report, obesity is a problem that costs $500 billion annually. The data shows that 63% of American women are overweight while 37% are obese.

In many developed countries such as the United States, obesity is an epidemic. The Centers for Disease Control and Prevention (CDC) estimates that in 2015–2016, 93.3 million (39.8 percent) American adults, and 13.7 million (18.5 percent) American children and teens were clinically obese.

Some of the causes of obesity are attributed to the present-day civilization that encourages indoor living and despises physical activity. They include:

- Living a sedentary lifestyle that allows for the accumulation of fats. In today's modern world, people use vehicles to move from one place to another as opposed to walking, or even cycling. Relaxation mainly involves watching movies or browsing the internet. As such, the energy generated from the food we eat is not utilized and is instead stored as fats.
- Diets that are rich in simple carbohydrates, fats, and calories. Eating large amounts of highly processed foods, fast foods, or sugary drinks leads to obesity because these foods contain high amounts of fats and calories.
- Inadequate sleep which may lead to hormonal changes which may leave you

craving foods that are rich in calories. In addition, inadequate sleep leads to the secretion of signal hormones such as ghrelin, which increases appetite, and leptin, which indicates when the body is satiated. This leads to increased food intake beyond the body's requirements.

- Genetics which have an impact on the metabolism rate, and how fat is stored. Children of obese parents are more likely to be obese than children of lean parents.
- Growing older. This leads to a decreased metabolic rate and less muscle mass, making it easier to gain weight.
- Medications. Some pharmaceutical drugs lead to weight loss as a side effect. Medication for diabetes, epilepsy, and psychotics, such as anti-depressants and medicines for schizophrenia, have been known to contribute to weight gain.
- Diseases such as: polycystic ovary syndrome, insulin resistance, Cushing's syndrome, and hypothyroidism. High insulin levels lead to increased insulin

resistance which implies that insulin is not absorbed by the cells in the body, but is instead stored as fat in the body, leading to obesity.

- Food addiction and aggressive marketing. Some junk and fast food producers are very aggressive in their marketing, sometimes making unhealthy food look healthy.

While the physical effects of obesity are widely documented and popularized, the psychological and emotional effects are often swept under the carpet, forgetting that patients suffering from obesity are also human.

We live in a society where slim and toned bodies are worshiped. Everything else is considered undesirable and unsightly. It then becomes easy for people suffering from obesity to suffer from anxiety and depression, and to lose their self-esteem and joy of life when society considers them to be undesirable. In extreme cases, this can lead to suicide.

However, by reading this book, you will discover

that obesity is not a death sentence. You will discover the use of intermittent fasting to shed off extra kilos in a sustainable manner. This is because intermittent fasting is not merely a short-term diet that promises you instant rewards. Instead, it is a way of life that guarantees you long-term results.

2.2 Reasons Why We Can't Afford to Ignore Obesity

As mentioned earlier, obesity is an epidemic in many developed and developing countries. The problem can no longer be ignored, nor can society turn a blind eye to it, because of the large number of people who are affected by this condition.

Not only does it lead to feelings of low self-esteem and depression, but obesity also robs society of important minds and personalities through suicide. A study that was published in the American Journal of Epidemiology states that people who are morbidly obese are five times more likely to experience suicidal thoughts as opposed to those who are not.

Obesity also creates conflict in romantic relationships. Studies indicate that obese partners are likely to carry feelings of shame and embarrassment concerning their food consumption and body weight. Any criticism regarding overeating habits may lead to arguments or conflict. This situation may be worse if a partner uses derogatory language to encourage the obese partner to hit the gym.

In addition, people with obesity are more likely to suffer from serious diseases and health conditions such as: cardiovascular disease, type 2 diabetes, hypertension, stroke, gallbladder disease, and osteoporosis, amongst other diseases.

2.3 Steps on how to Approach Obesity

Losing weight is a combination of a positive mindset, healthy eating, and exercises. You cannot achieve your weight loss goals if you ignore or overindulge in one aspect in the triad. To lose weight, an individual must first make peace with their current state and fully embrace who they are. Then, and only then, will they be able to witness real changes. In addition, you must be fully aware that losing weight will take a lot of time and effort. Most of all, you will need to make certain sacrifices and adjustments for your success.

Some of the steps you could put in place when approaching a weight loss journey are:

1. Set your goals: You will need to analyze your eating habits, current weight and any health conditions that you may have, and then create a game plan that will lead you to your goal. Inasmuch as losing weight is the ultimate goal, individuals should create smaller milestones to motivate them to move closer to that goal.

2. Surround yourself with positive energy: Avoid keeping the company of people who persistently remind you of your weight. Instead, surround yourself with people who are positive and encourage you to become your best self. For added motivation, you could join a slimming

club which is a great way to meet new people who share the same goals as you.

3. Make sure your goals are realistic and attainable: Remember that the journey of a thousand miles starts with a single step. It doesn't matter how small you start, just as long as you do start. This will provide you with a platform to work towards your goal.

4. Keep a track of all your activities: You could track yourself using a food diary, an exercise log, or a spreadsheet that contains both these records. By keeping track of your fitness exercises, eating habits, and even your moods, you become more accountable to yourself and thus, even more motivated to achieve your fitness goals.

5. Avoid stepping on the scale: For many people, the scale has been associated with negative and self-destructive thoughts. To avoid getting discouraged, don't bother stepping on the scale until you are at a point where you have

overcome the feelings that come with it. When at this point, make sure to weigh yourself frequently as studies show that people who weigh themselves more often are more likely to lose weight than those who do not.

6. Do not beat yourself up whenever you face minor set-backs or whenever you are unable to meet your goals. This will only serve to discourage you and will not help you to achieve your desired goal. Instead, take this set-back as an opportunity to get back on the drawing board to re-strategize.

7. Keep track of the sugars and starches in your diet: As mentioned earlier, over-consumption of foods and drinks that are rich in simple sugars and carbohydrates greatly contributes to obesity. It is therefore important to cut back on the amount of sugars and starches that you consume. In doing so, the body will have less glucose in the bloodstream and will instead burn down the fats stored in the

body to produce energy. You must therefore eat mindfully to effectively deal with the problem of obesity.

8. Eat plenty of proteins, fruits, and vegetables. Ideally, you should construct your meals such that you have a high protein source, a low-carb vegetable source, and a fat source. Your intake of carbohydrates should be within the daily recommended range of 20-30 grams. High protein diets have been proven to increase metabolism and to reduce cravings and frequent snacking. The fats that you consume should be healthy, so you have no reason to be afraid of fats.

9. Focus on eating whole and unprocessed foods as opposed to white foods. This is because white foods are highly processed with most of the essential nutrients being stripped away and replaced with synthetic vitamins. Whole foods on the other hand are healthier and more filling, reducing the occurrence of hunger pangs and cravings.

10. Drink plenty of unsweetened tea and coffee. This is because these drinks are believed to boost metabolism by 3% - 11%. In addition, they are very effective in suppressing cravings and feelings of hunger.
11. Avoid eating your foods hurriedly. People who eat very fast tend to gain more weight while those who eat slowly feel full, reducing the amount of food that they eat. In addition, eating slowly boosts the production of hormones that are known to reduce weight.
12. Take part in physical activities and exercises. This will help you to burn the calories and keep your body toned and fit. Generally, the degree of exercises varies from one person to the next. Based on age, health conditions, and weight loss goals, amongst many other factors, you could choose from low to medium to high-intensity exercises
13. Make sure you get adequate rest. Every night, you should be able to sleep for

eight hours, the daily recommended number. Poor and inadequate sleep is one of the reasons why people become obese.

Your Quick Start Action Step:
While it is universally agreed that losing weight is a difficult and sometimes a daunting task, preparation is the most critical part of the process which, when properly done, makes the whole process seem easier and less tasking.

As such, before starting your weight loss program, you should spend as much time as possible speaking to your doctor, researching online, preparing dietary plans and fitness exercises. These structures will be important in supporting you in the course of your journey, especially when you feel like giving up.

Once the preparation process is complete, you should then follow the steps which have been outlined above. Of course, the above-mentioned steps are not the Holy Grail to weight loss. As such, feel free to make any alterations and additions based on your personal needs and expectations.

If the dietary and fitness trials that you put into place do not work, do not be afraid to admit this to yourself. Do not look at them as failures, but rather as opportunities to learn and apply the acquired knowledge in the future.

Chapter 3: The Problem with our Diet

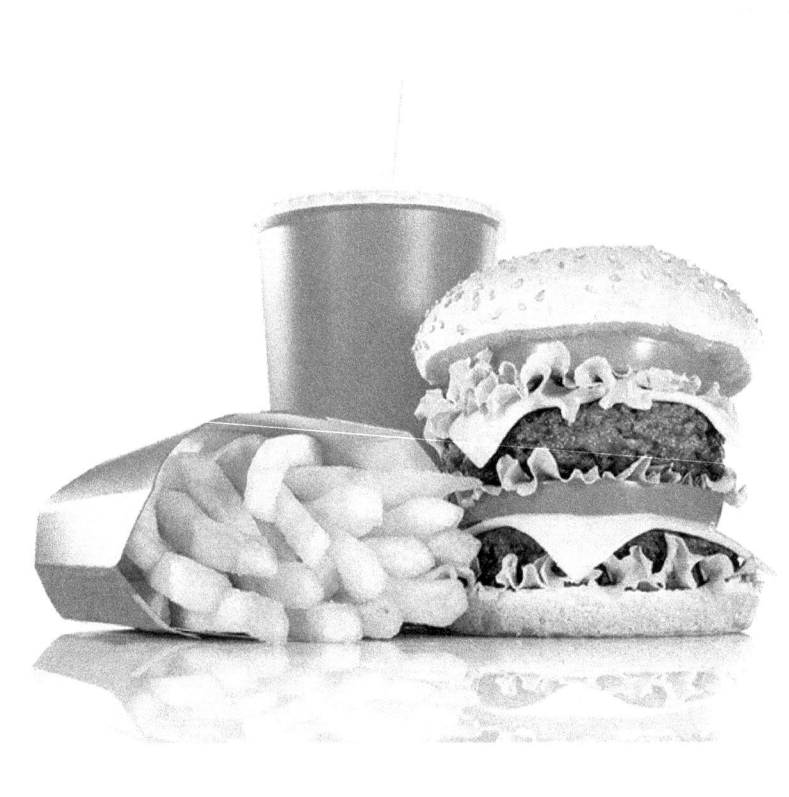

Chapter 3: The Problem with our Diet

3.1 Today's Fast Food Culture

Fast food culture began in the early 20th century with the discovery of the legendary hamburger which, at the time, was sold by the fast food chain restaurant, White Castle, and later, by the McDonald brothers. Today, there are hundreds, if not thousands of fast-food chain restaurants spread across the globe. Some of the most popular fast food restaurants include: Subway, McDonald's, Starbucks, Pizza Hut, Burger King, KFC, and Taco Bell, amongst many others.

The consumption of western-style fast food has spread widely throughout different cultures across the globe. Some of the popular fast food meals include: hamburgers, fries, fried chicken, fish, sandwiches, tacos, pizzas, hot dogs, onion rings, pitas, and ice cream. As such, the fast food industry makes billions of dollars annually and is a major employer of minimum wage workers in most developed countries.

Fast food restaurants are virtually located everywhere, from busy sidewalks and streets to airports, shopping centers, and even hospital lobbies. As such, fast foods are widely preferred due to the convenience that they offer. As opposed to spending time preparing meals, people can simply pop into the local fast food restaurant and grab a meal. Better still, one can simply order their meals from the comfort of their office or house.

Due to economies of scale, fast food is considerably cheaper compared to a traditional home-cooked meal. This factor has made the fast food culture spread widely, especially amongst the poor in America.

As a result, people who are exposed to fast foods have developed an unhealthy attachment to these foods to the extent that they are unable to fathom alternative meals and dietary plans.

3.2 Why is it Important to Shift to a Healthy Diet?

If not addressed, this problem has the potential of blowing up into a global catastrophe. Today,

2 out of every 3 American adults are obese. It is forecast that in the next 10 years, 75% of all adults in the United States will be obese. To prevent this, a paradigm shift in our dietary culture is paramount.

The truth of the matter is that people are unable to control what they eat. Due to the industrial nature of food production in these restaurants, consumers are not assured of the cleanliness standards that were upheld in preparing the food. In addition, the food is usually of lower quality, mainly because it is produced in bulk in large industrial kitchens where the focus is mainly on quantity as opposed to quality.

Since the beginning of the 20th century, there has been an upward trend in the cases of obesity, both within and outside America. It is no coincidence that this trend occurred at the same time as the advent of the fast food culture. It is a widely known fact that fast food is very fattening mainly because it involves the use of very greasy and fatty ingredients.

As if this is not enough, the growth of the fast food industry has been related to lifestyle diseases such as diabetes and cardiovascular disease. According to a report by the National Research Council, more than half of known cancers have been related to high-fat diets. This implies that most, if not all, lifestyle diseases can, to a large extent, be prevented.

3.3 The Paradigm Shift from Fast Food to Healthy Food

Today, few people in developed nations regard home-made food as a proper meal. Millennials are increasingly trying out new restaurants and eating joints, as opposed to trying out traditional food recipes, which ironically are widely available. Convincing such a generation to pursue healthier food options will therefore only take place through a serious paradigm shift that will greatly affect an industry which has been in operation for more than 50 years now.

Bearing in mind the magnitude of this problem, a shift from fast food to healthy food will call for a lot of time, effort and, most of all, dedication. You will first have to realize that fast food is not merely food but a culture, a way of life that is deeply engrained in our being. Hence, you will need to take one step at a time, realizing that if you make too many changes, you will most likely get discouraged, even before you start.

It is a generally accepted principle that you will need a month to affect each dietary change. However, the process could take less than the prescribed period, or considerably more. If it does take longer, do not look down upon yourself as people are inherently different and the expected results will be worth it.

Below are some steps that you could follow to change your diet:

1. Changing Beverages

The first step in shifting from an unhealthy to a healthy diet is changing the beverages that you consume. Drinks such as sodas and sweet teas are popularly referred to as liquid calories. This is because they contain little to no nutrients and instead have high amounts of calories. Overconsumption of these drinks leads to an increase in weight.

You could begin with a goal of eliminating liquid calories within a period of one month. This will be achieved by scaling down the quantity of liquid calories that you consume. Hence, if you drink more than two bottles a day, you could begin by scaling the quantity down by several bottles. If you do not drink water, or drink very little water, you could begin by consistently increasing your water intake until you achieve the daily recommended quantity of eight glasses per day. You could boost your water intake by adding lemon slices to your mineral water to make it a little more flavorful.

2. Boost your Intake of Fruits and Vegetables

Fruits and vegetables are an important constituent of a healthy diet. They are rich in nutrients, minerals, and phytonutrients, which boost the individual's immunity and help to fight disease-causing organisms.

To transition to a healthy diet, aim to increase your daily intake of fruits and vegetables to the daily recommended quantity of 4 to 5 cups within a period of one month. This can be achieved by including fruits and vegetables in all the three meals of the day, and any snacks that you consume in the course of the day. To boost your intake, you could steam some of the vegetables or incorporate some of the fruits in your foods.

It is important to note that there are many snacks and foods whose labels begin with the word "fruit" to make consumers believe that the products are healthy. However, most of the time, the fruits are not usually the main ingredient. As such, you should avoid such products and focus on eating the actual fruit.

3. Swap the Fats you Consume

Most, if not all fast food meals contain a lot of unhealthy oils which only serve to add several pounds to your weight. Commercially manufactured snacks and baked foods contain hydrogenated oils which are meant to extend the shelf lives of these products.

Red meats are believed to contain high amounts of saturated fats. These fats are believed to lead to heart diseases, diabetes, and colorectal cancer, one of the most common types of cancer.

To transition to a healthy diet, identify and eliminate all foods that contain both hydrogenated and partially hydrogenated oils. Replace the unhealthy oils with liquid oils such as olive, coconut, and canola oils, which are healthier. You could also increase your intake of healthier fats contained in avocados, olives, cold water fish, nuts, and seeds. In food preparation, avoid frying foods and opt for the healthier methods of food preparation such as baking and broiling.

Furthermore, you should reduce your intake of red meats and instead consume white meats such as chicken, fish, and turkey which contain less saturated fats and are therefore healthier.

4. Avoid Highly Refined Foods

The standard fast food meal, and by extension, the modern-day diet, is highly grained based. It contains foods such as rice, pasta, cereals, bread, biscuits, and crackers. These foods are highly refined and stripped of their most important nutrients and fibers. The nutrients are then replaced with synthetic vitamins and high fructose corn syrup. These carbohydrates are easily converted into glucose. Hence, over-eating these foods could easily result in increased weight and type 2 diabetes.

Transitioning to a healthier diet will involve foregoing some of these carbohydrates and opting for the healthier whole grain varieties. This implies that brown bread will replace white bread, and oatmeal will replace the sugary cereals that we have for breakfast.

Your Quick Start Action Step:

In addition to following the above-mentioned steps, maintaining a food diary is also very important in your journey to healthy eating. A food diary is a powerful tool that is used to track the food that you consume in order to understand your eating habits. This information is essential when making any dietary changes and in maintaining a healthy body weight. After all, knowledge is power!

To get the most out of your food diary, you need to be as truthful as possible. Cheating to look good will do you no good. Below are some of the things that you will need to keep a record of:

- The type of food, snack, or drink:

You should note down every meal that you consume, specifying whether there were any extras such as sauces, toppings, or condiments. This will be important in identifying the trends in your eating habits, if any.

- The quantity of foods and drinks:

Write down the amounts of food or drink that you consume. You could use different methods of measuring quantities including, but not limited to: volume, weight in grams or kilograms, and counting the number of items.

- The time and venue:

Make sure to note down the time in which you consume each meal as well as the place where you eat from, either the name of the restaurant or the specific room where you eat from.

- The person that you eat with:

You should specify whether you had any company as you were eating by listing down the names of the people you were eating with, if any.

- Activities engaged in:

List any activities that you took part in as you were eating. This could include watching the television, listening to the radio, playing games, working, or even holding a conversation.

- Your mood:

Most importantly, you must specify any emotions that you experienced as you were eating. This is important as it could help you to establish a relationship, if any, between your moods and your eating habits.

Chapter 4: Intermittent Fasting: An Overview on How to Lose Weight Faster

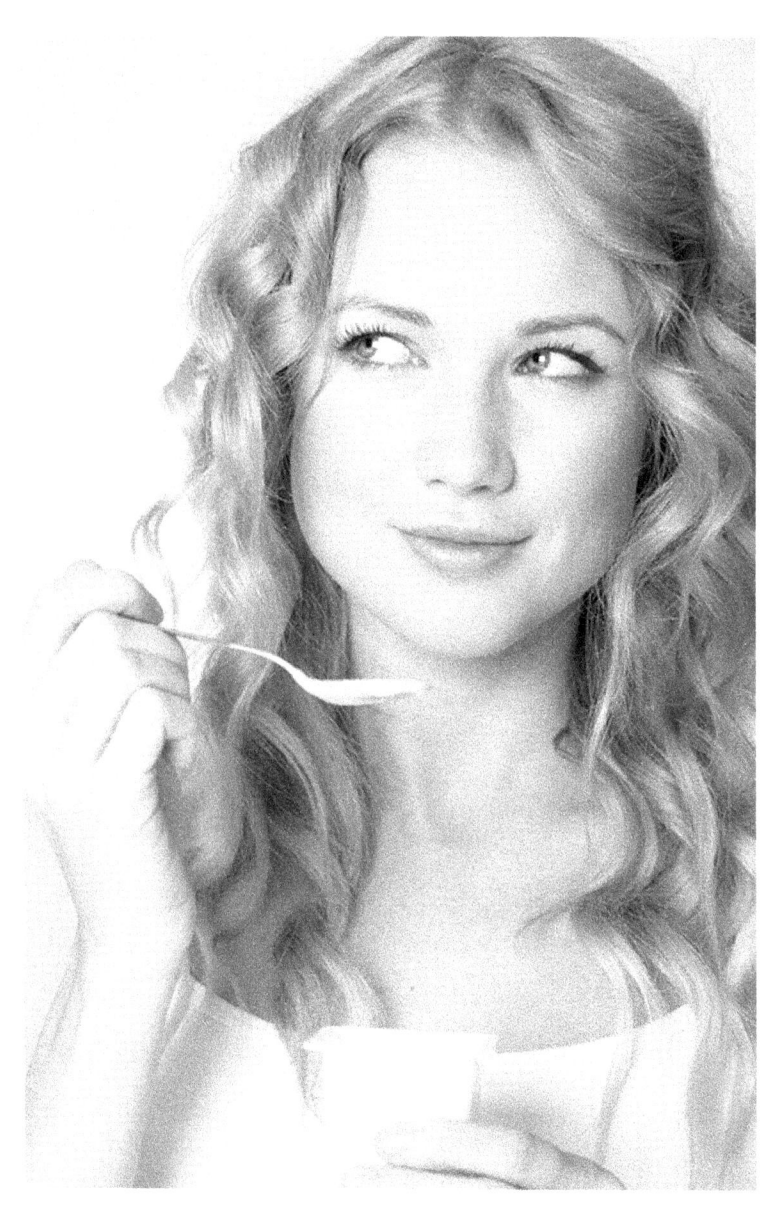

Chapter 4: Intermittent Fasting: An Overview on How to Lose Weight Faster

4.1 Expectations about the Intermittent Fasting Process

As mentioned earlier, the problem of obesity and being overweight is an issue that should be given priority in all nations across the world, with emphasis on developed nations that have adopted the western culture. Based on all the attention that this issue has been receiving, you could easily find yourself confused by the endless weight-loss strategies and dietary plans that are available in the market.

Each dietary plan and weight loss strategy is known to have its own benefits, and of course, challenges. However, none has proven to ensure efficient weight loss, while improving your longevity, as much as intermittent fasting has. As a result, the dietary plan has become very popular.

It is common practice that before you begin this dietary plan, you should visit a medical practitioner who will offer guidance on the best way to go about it. Generally, the diet is not recommended for pregnant women, women who are breastfeeding, or people with diabetes.

For those who are only beginning, the dietary plan can seem overwhelming and even impossible to some extent. There are numerous questions that you will want to ask, some of which do not have a straight answer, and which vary from one person to the next. However, we will try to shed some light on some of your burning questions.

The truth is that if you have been struggling with obesity or excessive weight, fasting can go a long way in helping you. However, you will need to keep in mind that intermittent fasting is not merely a dietary plan but a way of life. You will need to carefully plan your meals in advance depending on the method that you choose. Worse still is if you have a family, in which case you may need to have two separate meal plans.

To ensure the success of the diet, you will need to approach the whole process with a holistic view, realizing that eating a healthy diet and exercising are important pieces of the whole puzzle. You will have to avoid all junk foods and all foods rich in fats and calories or else you may find yourself gaining weight instead of losing it. In addition, to keep track of your progress you will need tools to measure or weigh yourself. These will include: a measuring scale, a tape measure, and possibly a weight tracking application. If you do not have access to any of these, you could monitor your visual progress by frequently taking photos of your body. You could also create a spreadsheet to keep track of your diet and the changes in your body over time.

Beginners should realize they may need a little help and motivation, especially on fast days. This implies that you may need to have a bottle of water on hand. If you have difficulties getting through your first few fast days, you could indulge in less than 500 calories. If you do consume more than 500 calories, then you will need to count this as an eating day. However, do not be discouraged, the process does get easier with time.

4.2 Benefits of the Overview on the Expectations of the Intermittent Fasting Process

The above overview is very important as it will guide you through the first few days or weeks of your dietary plan. It is also meant to save you the trouble of researching every single element of the intermittent fasting dietary plan by providing you with a conclusive starter pack and a companion that will walk you through the entire journey.

According to a study that was conducted and published in the Harvard School of Public Health, the drop-out rates of the subjects who were on the intermittent fasting diet were not significantly different from those subjects on calorie restricting diets. The range of drop-outs was between 0% and 65%, implying that intermittent fasting is not necessarily easier compared to other weight loss strategies and diets.

Bearing this in mind, it becomes important to seek the guidance of a specialist as the process may get extreme in some cases. In addition, despite the challenge that the diet possesses, be encouraged every step of the journey. Rest assured that with proper discipline, you will be able to achieve your weight loss goals.

4.3 Steps to Start the Intermittent Fasting Process

Daunting as the task may seem, you must always keep in mind that the journey of a thousand miles starts with a single step. Many are the times that people will experience food cravings and hunger pangs as soon as they get on the diet. However, do bear in mind that it gets easier!

Below are some of the steps that you will need to follow when starting and following the intermittent fasting diet:

1. Consult your medical practitioner before you start. This is especially the case if you suffer from any known medical

conditions, if you are pregnant, or if you are breastfeeding.

2. Decide on the intermittent fasting method that you would like to follow. As mentioned above, there are more than 7 types of intermittent fast. You must select the one that will work best for you and stick to it.

3. Keep it simple and easy. There are two possible ways that you could look at an intermittent fasting diet: a difficult and daunting duty that you owe to yourself, or simply as a self-experiment. In addition, you must break down the entire process into small and doable steps that will keep you motivated and on-track.

4. Identify the days of the week and schedule specific periods in the course of the day in which you will have your meals or fast. This will help to guide you through the process. However, the timings can always be changed depending on your schedule and bodily needs. In addition, identify a meal plan

that works. Ideally, the meal plan should be high in proteins, healthy fats, fruits, and vegetables. Carbohydrates should be consumed in moderation.

5. Zero in on the primary reason that you are fasting and work towards achieving the goal. Intermittent fasting does have a myriad of benefits for your body and you do need to zero in on one specific benefit for the best results.
6. During the intermittent fasting diet, make sure to drink the recommended eight glasses of water daily. In addition, avoid foods that are rich in fats, sugars, and refined carbohydrates even during your non-fasting days. This will consistently keep your body in the fat burning state.
7. Make sure to fit fasting into your life and not the other way around. The truth is that there will be moments where it will be impossible to fast during holidays, vacations, and other forms of celebration. Nonetheless, do not limit

your social interactions because of your fasting needs. Instead, take time off to celebrate with the greater community, and maybe later find a way to compensate.

8. Keep yourself busy. The one sure way to be positive that you do not feel the hunger is to keep yourself occupied. Often, you will be too busy to remember the hunger, as is the case during busy work days.
9. Ride the waves of hunger. It is scientifically proven that hunger pangs come in waves. In such moments, take a break and drink a cup of water, or a warm cup of coffee. This is because coffee is proven to be a mild appetite suppressant which will help you control your appetite.
10. Avoid snacking too much. Tempting as it may be to grab a snack during your feeding window, you must always bear in mind that small calories eventually add up. To solve this problem, make sure you set a strict calorie goal for yourself each

day, and correctly count your calories to make sure that you remain within this limit.

11. During eating days or periods, avoid binge eating or feasting. It is advised that you should pretend like nothing has happened and eat based on your dietary requirements. As mentioned, the meal should be nutritious and balanced.

12. Give yourself time to fully adapt to the intermittent fasting dietary plan. This could be anywhere between a week to a month. The duration greatly varies from one person to the next. However, if you take longer, take heart, do not be discouraged, we are all different. The most important thing is that you hit your goal.

13. Gradually increase your fasting with time. Once you are on the intermittent fasting diet, you could adjust your fasting based on your body and its response to intermittent fasting. Over time, you

could increase your fasting window from 14 hours to 16, or 20 hours.

14. Repeat the process. As mentioned, intermittent fasting is a way of life and you cannot expect the results to be visible within one day, one week, or even one month. The intended results will come with consistency in the pursuit of your goal.

15. Address any worries that you may have. The truth of the matter is that there are many questions that will come up in the course of the diet, some of which have answers, and some which do not. These questions have the potential of turning into worries which will make you nervous and unable to fully focus on your goal. Ergo, you should address any worries as soon as they come up. Always bear in mind that the intermittent fasting diet is not hazardous.

Your Quick Start Action Step:

To begin intermittent fasting, you must make sure that your mindset is right. Ensure that you are aware of the goal that you intend to achieve, the intermittent fasting method that you will use, and you are free of any anxiety or worries.

In addition, make sure to set aside at least 30 minutes each day to review your meal plan, clearly specifying the types of foods and drinks that you will have, if any, and the timing of your meals.

You must then follow each of the steps mentioned above and, where you have any questions, make sure to consult the advice of your doctor. Prepare a spreadsheet and record all changes frequently to keep track of your progress. If you feel sick or nauseated, stop the intermittent fasting diet immediately and ask for medical advice before continuing.

Chapter 5: Intermittent Fasting: Best Foods to Eat

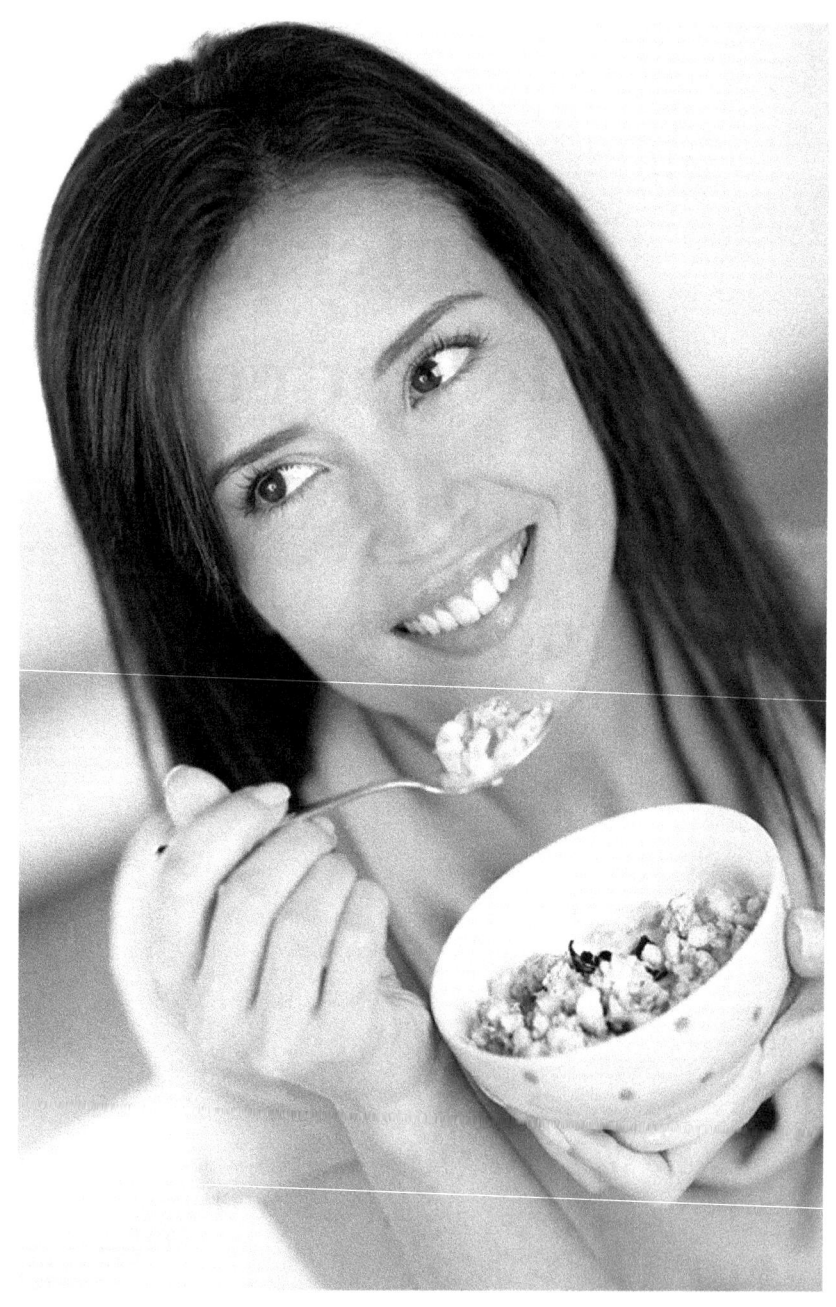

Chapter 5: Intermittent Fasting: Best Foods to Eat

5.1 What Type of Foods should be Considered for Intermittent Fasting?

Intermittent fasting, like many other dietary plans, involves the consumption of healthy and nutritious foods. The diet lays attention on both the quality and quantity of the foods that you consume to ensure that you achieve your desired goals.

Foods that are considered for intermittent fasting should contain all the important macro and micronutrients to contribute to good health and the general well-being of the person. Foods that are high in fiber are highly recommended for intermittent fasting diets. Fiber contained in foods is broadly classified as either soluble or insoluble fiber. However, both serve the functions of: contributing to satiety, regulating the speed of digestion, and by extension, the rate at which glucose is absorbed into the bloodstream, reducing constipation and the risk of colon cancer. Fiber rich vegetables include: broccoli, cucumbers, carrots, Brussel sprouts, beetroots, spinach, kale, and celery roots, amongst others.

Foods that are rich in proteins are also highly recommended. High protein diets are important as they reduce your appetite, cravings and hunger levels, boost your metabolism and fat burning, contribute to increased muscles, and are generally good for your bones. The proteins that you consume should be low carb, and in the case of meats, lean. This is because fatty cuts of beef or pork usually contain saturated fats, which are essentially unhealthy, and could lead to increased cholesterol levels.

Fruits and vegetables are also of particular importance. Vegetables are known to contain fibers which take a long time to be digested in the gut. As such, these vegetables create a feeling of satiation, keeping hunger pangs and cravings at bay. Fruits on the other hand are rich in minerals and vitamins, which boost your general body immunity and contribute to your wellbeing.

People are advised to avoid foods that are rich in saturated fats, refined sugars, and simple carbohydrates. These include: red meats, white foods, and all foods that are prepared through deep-frying.

5.2 Why are these Foods Important in Achieving your Intermittent Fasting Goals

Eating foods that are rich in both macro and micronutrients are very important in maintaining the health and general wellbeing of the human body. In addition, while starvation is essentially the deprivation of food and important nutrients, intermittent fasting is simply a cycle of feeding and fasting. As such, the foods consumed during the feeding window should be highly nutritious or else the intermittent fasting diet will not work. Nutrients are also important in ensuring that the biological process of autophagy is operational. Autophagy refers to the process by which the cells in the body can remove any junk in the bloodstream and recycle wastes. Malnourishment causes the autophagy process to slow down and may cause the cells to cannibalize and result in fast aging,

Foods that are rich in fiber have numerous benefits for people who are fasting intermittently. First, foods that are rich in fiber are important in preventing constipation. This is because soluble fibers absorb a lot of water, making your stool softer and larger, while insoluble fibers make your stool bulkier. As such, the stool is easily able to pass through your gut, preventing the constipated feeling. Second, foods that are rich in fiber absorb a lot of water in the gut. They are then converted into a gel which makes the process of digestion take a longer time. This in turn has the effect of making you feel satiated for longer periods of time. Satiation then reduces the occurrence of any hunger pangs and cravings, making it easier to fast for longer periods of time.

Foods that are rich in protein are also important in contributing towards building muscle and lean tissue. Proteins contain amino acids which are important building blocks for the body. This implies that the muscles and the cells in the body require proteins to remain healthy. Hence, proteins allow you to lose weight while still maintaining some body mass. Proteins also create a feeling of satiation which allows you to go for extended periods of time without breaking your fast.

Eating a diet that is rich in vegetables is also very important since vegetables are low in fat and calories, reducing the occurrence of heart diseases. They are also important sources of nutrients which contribute to your general health. Vegetables also contain fibers, which as we have mentioned, creates a feeling of satiation and reduces constipation.

5.3 Best Foods to Try for Intermittent Fasting

1. Vegetables are some of the important foods that you will need during your intermittent fast. This is because they contain plenty of nutrients, including but not limited to: vitamin C, vitamin A, vitamin D, sodium, magnesium, potassium, and folic acid.

Potassium may lower your blood pressure, decrease the chances of developing kidney stones, and reduce your bone loss. Most importantly, vegetables are low in fats and calories, which is important in your weight loss journey. Some of the common vegetables that you could add to your diet include: carrots, cabbage, cauliflower, broccoli, beetroot, spinach, kale, bell peppers, and lettuce, amongst others.

2. Like vegetables, fruits also have a myriad of benefits for your health. They contain nutrients such as: calcium, fiber, iron, magnesium, potassium, sodium, vitamin A, vitamin C, iron, and folate, amongst others. These nutrients are very important in building up the body's immunity for protection against disease-causing germs and bacteria. In addition, they are also low in fats and calories. Some of these fruits include: oranges, tangerines, lime, apples, bananas, pineapples, mangoes, blueberries, strawberries, peaches, and grapes, amongst others. A recent study has revealed that

berries are rich in flavonoids, which result in smaller increases in BMI over a 14-year period.
3. Foods that are rich in proteins are also known as body-building foods mainly because they contain important amino acids which form the building blocks of our muscles and cellular structure. Some common foods that are rich in protein and suitable for the intermittent fasting diet include: chicken breast, eggs, tofu, mushroom, lean cuts of beef, pork and lamb, legumes such as beans, peas, chickpeas, and lentils.
4. Nuts and seeds provide numerous fats, fibers, vitamins, and minerals. Some of the nutrients include: vitamin E, calcium, zinc, potassium, magnesium, manganese, and copper, amongst others. Nuts contain lots of healthy fats which create a feeling of satiation, which helps to reduce appetite and hunger. Furthermore, studies seem to suggest that consuming about 30 grams of nuts daily may reduce the risk of developing

heart diseases, as well as your cholesterol levels. The fibers in nuts and seeds also reduce the reabsorption of cholesterol into the gut. Some of the recommended nuts and seeds include: almonds, walnuts, pistachios, macadamia, pumpkin seeds, sunflower seeds, and watermelon seeds.

5. Whole foods are also highly recommended for the intermittent fasting diet, and more generally as part of a healthy diet. This is because they are rich in dietary fibers and B vitamins. Dietary fibers are important for healthy bowel movements, and to reduce constipation. B vitamins are also important to release fats, proteins, and carbohydrates. Generally, whole foods are important in reducing cholesterol levels and the risk of heart diseases. Some of the whole foods that are recommended for the intermittent fasting diet include: oats, quinoa, sorghum, barley, and white rice.

6. Unsaturated fats and oils are also highly recommended for the intermittent fasting diet. The fats and oils are healthy and

contribute to the feeling of satiation, which is important if you are going to be fasting for extended periods of time. Some of the common sources of healthy fats and oils include: olive oil, coconut oil, peanut butter, almond butter, and sunflower butter, amongst others.

Your Quick Start Action Step:
Before starting the intermittent fasting diet, you should check your pantry and refrigerator to make sure that you have some of these foods and the ingredients that will be required to make a meal that is in line with the intermittent fasting diet. If you do not have some of these foods, make sure to visit your local grocery store to stock your pantry.

Chapter 6: Intermittent Fasting: Best Time to Eat in a Day

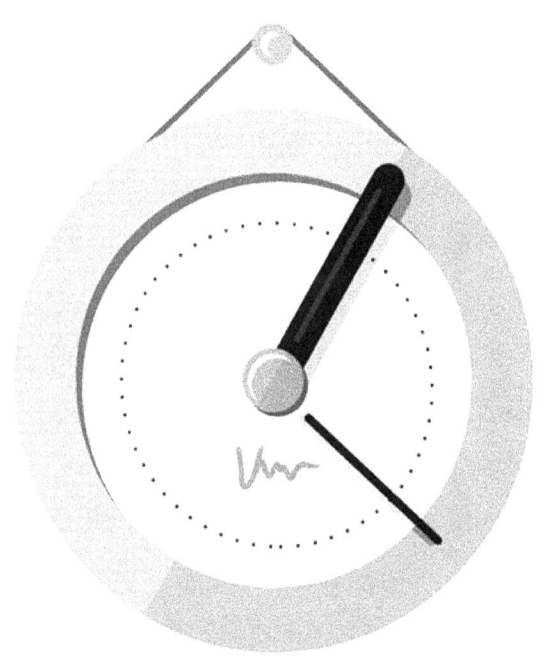

Chapter 6: Intermittent Fasting: Best Time to Eat in a Day

6.1 The Relevance of the Time of Day when Intermittent Fasting

It is a widely shared opinion that it does not matter what time of day you decide to eat. What matters most in determining whether you gain or lose weight is the type, amount of food, and the amount of physical activity that you engage in during the day. As accurate as this may sound, it is sadly a myth, one that has become widely popularized over time.

The truth of the matter is that the time of day is extremely important in determining the success of your intermittent fast. Many folks will advise you against eating large meals in the evening, stating that you will not get the opportunity to burn off the food, causing it to be stored in the body as fat. While this may not be true in the strict sense, there is evidence that links obesity to feeding on heavy meals at night.

The best time to have your eating window, and by extension, the largest meal of the day, is any time between noon and 3:00 pm. People who finish their calories for the day by 3:00 pm have improved insulin sensitivity, lower blood pressure, and reduced hunger pangs and cravings.

This approach is effective because the body follows a natural circadian rhythm in which it burns fuel during the day, then enters storage mode during the night. As such, when people finish their calories by 3:00 pm, they will have burnt glucose and fat during the day and there will be no fats to be stored in the body at night.

In addition, the natural circadian rhythm of the ghrelin hormone leads to increased hunger at night. Having your last meal by 3:00 pm therefore becomes beneficial, as it prevents people from consuming excessive calories, especially at night, when people find it most difficult to control their food intake due to increased hunger.

Limiting our feeding to these hours is extremely beneficial as we can control our blood pressure and blood sugar. Our hormonal control becomes better leading to improved disease prevention and reduced inflammation in the body. In addition, you will sleep better as you will go to bed with little hunger. This will reduce the occurrence of stomach upsets, heartburns, and feelings of being too full, which are associated with poor sleeping patterns.

6.2 The Rationale Behind Time of Day

- The human body, like the bodies of other animals, has been scientifically proven to operate in circadian rhythms. These are cyclical changes in behavior and hormones which occur every 24 hours.
- The circadian rhythms govern all hormones, including but not limited to: growth hormones, parathyroid hormones, insulin, and ghrelin. Of importance in this case is insulin, which is proven to contribute to weight gain, and ghrelin, which is a hormone that controls hunger.

- Ghrelin rises and falls based on the natural circadian rhythm. Hunger, which is controlled by the ghrelin hormone, also rises and falls based on the natural circadian rhythm. The ghrelin hormone is usually lowest early in the morning, at about 8:00 am and highest later in the evening at about 8:00 pm.
- Correspondingly, hunger is lowest early in the morning at about 7:50 am and highest in the evening at around 7:50 pm. Hence, we see that hormones are key in the regulation of hunger.
- At 7:50 am, hunger is low. It therefore makes no sense to force ourselves to feed. At 7:50 pm, hunger is maximally stimulated, implying that the more food you consume, the higher the insulin levels in your bloodstream, and the greater the weight gain.
- Since the hormonal regulation of hunger is independent of the fast/eat cycle in an intermittent fasting diet, it becomes important to establish an optimal

strategy that will determine the best time to have the largest meal of the day.
- Bearing this in mind, the optimal strategy becomes eating the largest meal between noon and 3:00 pm. Hence, implying that individuals on an intermittent fasting diet should schedule their eating windows during this time.

6.3 Steps to Follow

It is true that the concept of a limited feeding period with prolonged periods of fasting may terrify you greatly. To you, the concept of fasting may be synonymous to starvation and may invoke feelings of suffering and anguish. Worse still, you probably cannot fathom why you should avoid eating food. Yet it is right there, tempting you to eat it. The idea of going a whole day without food may even be incomprehensible to you.

However, I assure you that the intermittent fasting diet is indeed doable. This method, for lack of a better word, could be referred to as the 21/3 method. In this method, you get to fast for a period of 24 hours and only get to eat food in a 3-hour window between noon and 3:00 pm. The method could also be applied during alternate-day fasting.

Below are the steps to follow when implementing an intermittent fasting diet where the feeding window is optimally scheduled between noon and 3:00 pm:

1. On the day that you choose to begin your intermittent fasting diet, enjoy your last meal of the day between noon and 3:00 pm. After this meal, you will begin calculating your fasting hours beginning from 3:00 pm.
2. Proceed with your day, only drinking water, unsweetened tea, and coffee whenever you experience a pang of hunger. When the night falls and evening comes, make sure to sleep for 8 hours. By the time you wake up, you will have completed more than half of your fasting period.
3. If you really cannot make it until morning, it is highly recommended that

you consume a light meal that is high in protein, such as a protein shake or a few carbs. This meal is best eaten at least one hour before you go to bed. It is important as it will supply you with all the important nutrients while keeping your stomach full and free of hunger or cravings.

4. Based on the natural circadian rhythm of the human body, you are less likely to feel hungry in the morning. In addition, if you had a proper meal the previous day, the chances of feeling hungry are even lower. However, you can always drink some mineral water, unsweetened tea, or coffee if you do experience any hunger. If you really cannot make it to noon, you can have a smoothie or a light meal to break your fast. However, if you can take it, push yourself to noon without eating any solid food.

Your Quick Start Action Step:

Having gone through the above steps, I believe that you are confident that you can implement the intermittent fasting diet above. You will need to have prepared a dietary plan in advance, which you will use to dictate the meals that you have during these periods. The meals will need to be rich in proteins, fruits and vegetables, and low in carbohydrates, as per the intermittent fasting diet.

The final and most important thing will then be to schedule a time between noon and 3:00 pm to have your meals. While having your meals, avoid eating in a hurry, as you will be more likely to over-eat. Eating slowly creates a feeling of fullness in your stomach, which limits the amount of food that you consume.

However, to ensure the success of this intermittent fasting diet, you must let go of the notion that has long been embedded in us that dinner is the most important meal of the day. You will need to reprogram your thinking, which, though difficult, is very possible. With reduced pressure to prepare a large meal for dinner, you will have more time to yourself to spend on other activities that equally need your attention.

While our social needs and demands may make it difficult to have the last meal of the day before 3:00 pm, you must always believe that where there is a will, there is a way. In addition, you must remember that the intermittent fasting diet is meant to fit into your life and not the other way around. Hence, do not restrict your social interactions based on this diet. First enjoy yourself, then later strategize on how to compensate.

Chapter 7: Picking the Right Meal Plan

FRUITS
Let fruits jazz up your feast!

- ☐ Apples
- ☐ Avocado
- ☐ Bananas
- ☐ Blueberries
- ☐ Cranberries

Chapter 7: Picking the Right Meal Plan

7.1 Picking the Right Meal Plan

Now that you have heard all about the intermittent fasting diet, all that remains is learning about how you can prepare a seven-day meal plan. Depending on the method of intermittent fasting that you follow, there are different foods and drinks that you could combine to form a unique meal plan that will suit your dietary needs. In this case, we will focus on the 16/8 method that involves restricting the hours in which you can eat.

It is medically recommended that the meal plan should contain several small meals and snacks which are evenly spread out within the eating window. The meal plan should not allow for binge eating or feasting but should control the portions of food and snacks that one eats at each point in time, depending on the level of hunger. To maximize the potential health benefits and to ensure weight loss, it is important to stick to a nutritious diet. You should avoid all manner of junk foods, foods that are rich in sugar and simple carbohydrates, and all white and refined foods.

Ideally, the best meal plan should contain: foods that are rich in soluble fibers such as nuts, beans, fruits, and vegetables. Foods that are rich in protein such as meat, fish, nuts and tofu, whole grains such as oats, barley, quinoa, and buckwheat, vegetables such as broccoli, cauliflower, cucumbers, and tomatoes. Also, foods that are rich in healthy fats and oils such as nuts, seeds, and even fish.

The meal plan should also include beverages that are free of calories, such as mineral water, unsweetened teas and coffees, or cinnamon teas.

7.2 The Importance of Picking the Right Meal Plan

The right meal plan should consist of small meals and snacks that are spread out during the eating period. This is important in keeping hunger under control by preventing excessive hunger pangs. The prevention of excessive hunger pangs also reduces the likelihood of binge eating and feasting.

In addition, due to the small, but high, frequency of the meals, the blood sugar levels are maintained at a relatively constant level, preventing the occurrence of insulin resistance or high blood pressure.

The right meal plan should be nutritious for the success of the intermittent fasting diet. Nutritious meals contain all the important proteins, carbohydrates, vitamins, and minerals for the healthy development of the person. Any meal plan that is not nutritious is more likely to lead to weight gain than it is likely to lead to weight loss.

The presence of soluble fibers in a meal plan is important, especially during intermittent fasting as it creates a feeling of being full, preventing any hunger pangs that may occur. During digestion, the soluble fibers attract a lot of water, turning into gel and slowing down the digestion process, hence creating the feeling of being full.

Foods that are rich in protein are also important, as they provide the body's muscles with all the protein nutrients that are required for healthy growth, while keeping the stomach full and preventing hunger pangs.

The right meal plan should also contain whole foods, as opposed to white foods. This is because white foods are highly refined and contain synthetic vitamins, while whole foods are not refined, contain no synthetic vitamins, and are therefore highly nutritious.

Calorie-free drinks such as water are important as they are not only used to remain hydrated, but also to control hunger and appetite for food. Black unsweetened coffee is particularly important, as it boosts the metabolism of the body, increasing the rate at which glucose and fats are turned into energy.

Raw fruits and vegetables are particularly important, as they contain the soluble fibers which create a feeling of being full. In addition, they contain important vitamins and minerals, which are utilized by the body to boost its immunity.

7.3 Steps on Picking the Right Meal Plan

While using the 16/8 method of intermittent fasting, you will need to schedule an eight-hour eating period at a time of your own choosing. However, you should keep in mind that the optimal time to eat is usually between noon and 3:00 pm in line with the natural circadian rhythm.

Below are some of the steps that you will need to follow to identify the right meal plan:

1. Ideally, you should begin your day without any carbohydrates in your system. This is done to ensure that the body is in a state of ketosis where it is burning fats to produce energy rather than glucose.
2. The meals of the day should be spread out across the 8-hour period depending on the dietary needs, hunger, and the activities that you will engage in at a particular point in time. For example, you could divide the feeding window into

3 distinct meal plans which are equally spaced out.
3. In addition, you could consume coffee every morning to boost your metabolism, reduce your appetite, and give you a positive mood and stamina. The daily recommended amount of coffee that you can consume within a day is 2 – 3 small cups. You could drink coffee during your fasting window to reduce any hunger pangs that you may experience.
4. You should have the first meal of the day within 3 – 4 hours after waking up. Pushing this meal later into the day forces the body to burn up some of its fat reserves to generate energy without relying on glucose from food. You should have the last meal of the day 3 – 4 hours before you retire to bed. Based on the natural circadian rhythm of the ghrelin hormone, this ensures that you do not eat food at a point in which the body is storing up its reserves as it might lead to weight gain.

5. The first meal of the day, which is meant to break the fast, is supposed to be very healthy and modest in size. Breaking the fast with a very large meal or through binge eating will slow down the fat burning process in your body, making you tired in the late hours of the morning. The first meal should contain 300 – 400 calories and should generally contain some protein, healthy fats, and fruits. Some of the foods that you could eat at this point include: canned tuna, an omelet, chicken breast, berries, apples, avocados, almond milk, protein shakes, and some almond nuts.
6. Your second and third meals of the day should each contain about 500 – 600 calories and should be high in protein and with moderate amounts of fats and carbohydrates. An example of such a meal would be: chicken breast, some yam wedges, veggies, and blueberries.
7. You should always keep in mind that intermittent fasting is a dietary plan that

restricts your eating to certain periods in the course of the day or the week. Hence, if you successfully complete your fasting period but consume twice, or thrice, the amount of food and calories that you are supposed to, your fast will essentially be pointless and could result in weight gain and feelings of fatigue. Hence, both food quality, and food quantity, must be honored.

8. All meals that you consume should contain healthy portions of both soluble and insoluble fibers. This is because fibers quickly absorb water once they enter the digestive system. They then turn into gel, which is digested slowly, creating a feeling of fullness. In addition, fiber does reduce constipation. Fiber is mainly contained in foods such as broccoli, cauliflower, and Brussels sprouts.

9. Berries are also an important addition to your meal plan. They are believed to contain healthy portions of vital vitamins

and nutrients, which boost your immunity and contribute to your general wellbeing. It is scientifically proven that people who consume healthy portions of strawberries and blueberries experience smaller increases in BMI over a 14-year period.

10. Any snacks that you consume should not contain carbohydrates. They should mainly include coffee, green tea, apples, or even some nuts.

11. Fish is highly recommended as it contains healthy fats, proteins, and vitamin D. Because of this, fish has long been considered a 'brain food', as it highly nourishes the body and, by extension, the brain.

12. Probiotics are also important constituents of your meal plan. The enzymes and bacteria in the body thrive on consistency and diversity. Hence, when you feel hungry, you may experience some side effects, such as constipation. Probiotic rich foods and

supplements are therefore important in ensuring that the enzymes and bacteria responsible for digestion are satisfied, preventing any side effects.

13. Once you have identified your fasting and feeding windows, you should try to keep these periods constant, since hunger is controlled by the ghrelin hormone, which follows the circadian cycle. Hence, after some weeks, you will realize that you will experience hunger at specific points in time, and it is best to maintain this regular pattern.
14. Leguminous plants are also very important in your intermittent fasting diet. Legumes such as beans, peas, chickpeas, lentils, and even black beans, are low-calorie carbohydrates which are very important in your intermittent fasting diet.
15. While preparing a meal plan, some of the foods that you should avoid at all costs include: refined starches, white foods,

added sugars, trans fats, and processed foods.

Your Quick Start Action Step:
Coming up with a meal plan that is suited to the intermittent fasting diet is a process that will require you to schedule significant amounts of time to conduct in depth research, to consult with your doctor, and to source for all the materials that you need.

You should keep in mind that the foods that you include in your meal plan should be low-calorie and nutrient-dense foods that will nourish your muscles and organs, while allowing your body to burn down fats to release energy. It may be difficult to list down all the foods that you can eat, however, as a general guideline, you should focus on: lean proteins, plant proteins, fruits, vegetables, nuts, and seeds.

The key to losing weight, therefore, involves a healthy and well-balanced diet that ensures constant energy levels for the body to carry out its normal functions. Most importantly, consistency and sticking to the diet is important for the intermittent fasting diet to be successful. As a disclaimer, if your meal plan makes you dizzy or weak, you are advised to terminate the meal plan immediately, and to seek the guidance of a nutritionist or a medical practitioner.

Chapter 8: The One Meal a Day Approach

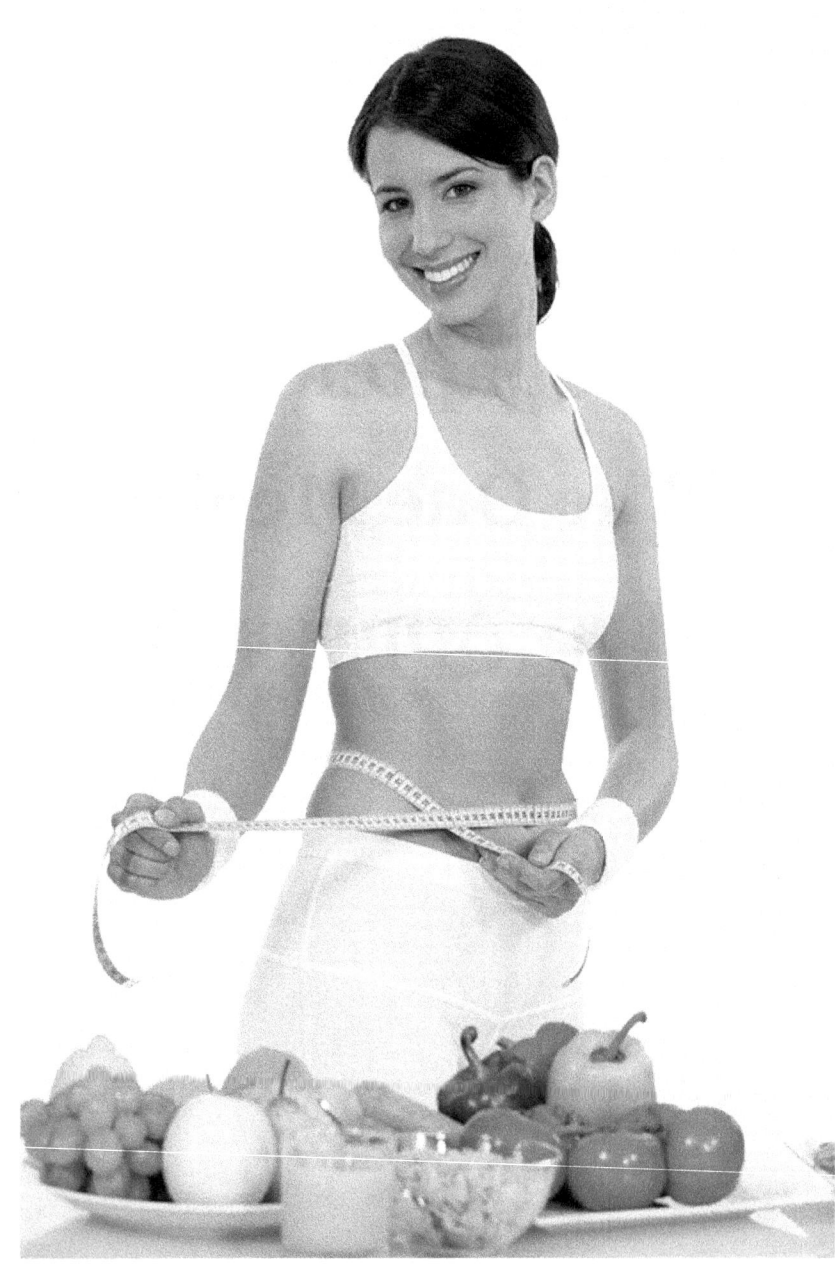

Chapter 8: The One Meal a Day Approach

8.1 Background Information

Today, intermittent fasting is one of the most powerful tools that you could use to optimize your anatomy and biology, while still shedding off some extra pounds. The methods of intermittent fasting range from calorie restriction in the course of the day, to alternating between regular feeding days and fasting days, to limiting the number of hours that you get to eat within the day.

The One Meal a Day Approach (OMAD) is a form of intermittent fasting in which you get to fast for a 23-hour window and get to eat during a one hour feeding window every single day. Unlike the other methods of intermittent fasting, OMAD shrinks the feeding window even further. As such, the method is not suitable for beginners, as it is an extreme form of intermittent fasting, or the Warrior Diet method of intermittent fasting.

The diet is based on the principles of calorie restriction and consuming low-calorie diets during one particular time of the day or night. This then allows you to fast for the remaining 23 hours of the day. The body is then able to burn up the fat reserves to produce energy, consequently leading to weight loss. Any carbohydrates or fruit sugars that are consumed during the feeding window then help in fat mobilization.

The OMAD allows you to gain all the benefits of an intermittent fasting diet, while greatly simplifying your daily schedule. This is because, unlike the conventional 3 meal per day approach, you will spend less time in meal planning and preparation, giving you time to engage in other activities.

Most dieters will have their feeding window during dinner time, since it is at this time that we experience maximum hunger, in line with the natural circadian rhythm of the ghrelin hormone. In addition, you could have unsweetened black coffee or tea in the course of the day to take care of any hunger pangs, and to suppress your appetite. You could also have an apple or an egg during the day.

8.2 Why does the OMAD Method Work?

The OMAD is considered to be an unconventional method of losing weight. The idea of having one meal per day is considered excessive and unnecessary. Hence, many people cringe at the idea of the OMAD.

However, before you make your conclusion and dismiss the diet, the proponents of OMAD highlight several benefits that are associated with this approach.

From an evolutionary standpoint, human beings engaged in food-seeking activities, which would last anywhere from a couple of hours to a few days. Human beings then developed powerful mechanisms and adaptations which allowed their bodies, and by extension, brains, to function at their optimal levels despite the scarcity in food.

The mechanisms that allowed humans to survive such periods of fasting are believed to have numerous benefits, which have been negated by the present-day sedentary lifestyle characterized by continuous and abundant food supply.

Through the OMAD, the body is supercharged by activating the stress response pathways, which boost mitochondrial performance, the body's metabolism, the production of hormones (such as growth hormones), the repair of DNA in your cells, and prevent the occurrence of chronic diseases such as: diabetes, high blood pressure, and insulin resistance. In addition, OMAD activates autophagy, the mechanism that the body uses to clean up damaged cells, toxins, and wastes.

As mentioned above, the OMAD provides for one meal each day. This implies that the intake of calories is generally very restricted compared to other individuals who eat throughout the day. Furthermore, it becomes impossible for one to have a surplus of calories, even when consuming unhealthy foods. Hence, the approach is very efficient in weight loss.

In addition, many people who follow the conventional 'three meals a day' approach can attest to the sluggish feeling that one experiences after having their lunch. As the digestion process proceeds, people experience a groggy feeling, slowing down their general productivity. Hence, the proponents of this method believe that the approach eliminates the sluggishness that people experience in the afternoon.

8.3 Steps to Follow When Doing the OMAD Approach

The OMAD approach can be very tasking, to say the least. You will need a lot of effort, discipline, and commitment if you are to succeed in this method of intermittent fasting. In addition, avoiding food for 23 hours straight will require you to reprogram your thinking away from the typical 'three meals per day' approach.

Below are some of the steps that you will need to follow to get onto the OMAD approach:

1. Consult your medical practitioner before you start. This is especially the case if you suffer from any known medical

conditions, if you are pregnant, or if you are breastfeeding.

2. Identify the primary reason that you are fasting using the OMAD approach, and work towards achieving that goal. Intermittent fasting does have a myriad of benefits for your body and you do need to zero in on one specific benefit for the best results.

3. Identify and schedule the one hour that will form your feeding window. The optimal feeding window is scientifically proven to be between noon and 3:00 pm, based on the natural circadian rhythm. However, you could also schedule your one-hour feeding window in the evening, such that it coincides with dinner time, the time in which we experience the most hunger. Regardless of the window that you select, consistency is key.

4. Take one step at a time. The truth of the matter is that the OMAD approach is not as easy as the snap of a finger. You will need to slowly ease into the OMAD diet

at your own pace. It is recommended that you break down the entire process into small and doable steps, which will keep you highly motivated. Since people are inherently different, it is also likely that different people will take different durations of time to fully transition into the OMAD diet. Despite this, be encouraged to run your own race. After all, what matters is that you eventually achieve your goal.

5. Cut down on the amount of carbohydrates that you consume. When you eat lots of carbohydrates and starches, you increase the amount of glucose that is released into the bloodstream. Any excess glucose will then be converted into glycogen and stored in the liver. As such, it will take a long period of time for the body to fully shift to the fat-burning mode which is required for weight loss. In addition, a low-carb diet will keep you satisfied for longer, while reducing your appetite, and

the crankiness that is associated with foods that are rich in starch.

6. Because of the extreme calorie restriction under the OMAD diet, you can virtually eat unhealthy foods, and your calorie intake will still be way below that of a person who eats three meals a day. To many people, this implies that you can eat anything you want. However, it is important to note that just because you can eat anything does not mean that you should. Your meal will still need to be well-balanced, and nutritious enough to contribute to your good health and general wellbeing.

7. Some of the meals that you should focus on eating include, but are not limited to: plant proteins, lean meats, eggs, dairy products, nuts, seeds, healthy fats and oils, whole foods, and different herbs and spices. The main foods that you should avoid include: white refined foods, cashew nuts, fatty meats, vegetable oil,

butter, margarine, mayonnaise, soft drinks, and energy drinks.

8. The perfect meal plan should therefore contain, but is not limited to: at least five types of vegetables, three types of fruits, lean meats, unsalted nuts, buttermilk to aid in digestion, dark chocolate, and mineral water to remain hydrated. The meal plan should contain a wide range of both macro and micronutrients to keep your body fully nourished. Feeding on one nutrient will therefore do you no good.

9. When you initially begin the OMAD diet, you will not have the physical or mental energy to work out because of the long fasting hours. However, you could still engage in light stretching exercises and yoga sessions to keep your muscles active. Once you get the hang of the intermittent fasting diet, you could include toning exercises to keep your skin from sagging. Alternatively, you

could consult a fitness expert to structure a weight loss program for you.

10. It can be argued that the most important aspect of effecting the OMAD diet is developing the discipline and willpower to stick to the diet despite the cravings and hunger pangs that you are likely to experience. This is because hunger is a powerful feeling that can demotivate and disorient you. You will need to overcome the habit of having three meals per day by persistently convincing yourself that you can do it.

Your Quick Start Action Step:

Schedule some time to carry out in depth research and to consult a medical practitioner to provide you with all the knowledge that you will need before starting the OMAD diet. This is especially so if you are suffering from any known medical condition, if you are pregnant, or breastfeeding.

Armed with the necessary knowledge, you could follow the steps highlighted above to come up with the timing of your feeding window, a suitable meal plan, and any workouts that you plan to engage in. You will need to go out and shop for some of these foods and ingredients to restock your refrigerator and kitchen cabinets.

As you pursue this journey, you will need to realize that it will test your will and determination countless times. Hence, you will need to constantly motivate yourself and keep the company of positive people, preferably people who are pursuing the same goal. You could also frequently track your progress by recording it in a spreadsheet.

If you feel weak, dizzy, sluggish, constantly tired, or experience some brain fog, you may need to stop the OMAD diet and seek the advice of your medical practitioner. You will need to realize that all bodies are fundamentally different, and you could still achieve your intended goals with a mild form of intermittent fasting.

Nonetheless, the OMAD diet is an effective diet mainly because it helps you to prevent any future weight gain.

Chapter 9:
Healthy Recipes

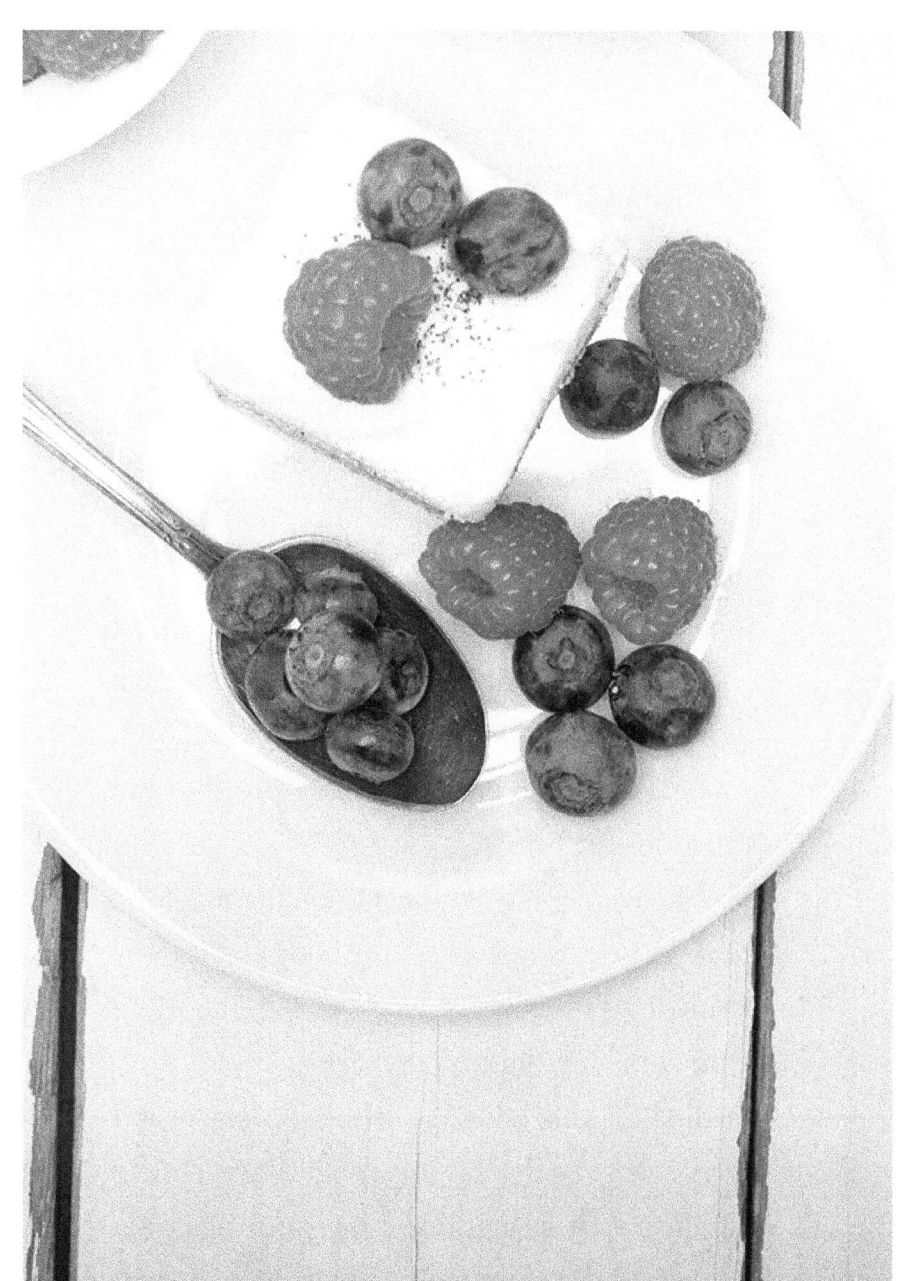

Chapter 9: Healthy Recipes

9.1 Healthy Recipes During Intermittent Fasting

Intermittent fasting has everything to do with calorie restriction just as much as it has everything to do with restricting the hours in which an individual can consume meals. As such, food quality is just as important as food quantity.

Successful weight loss using the intermittent fasting diet necessitates the use of a three-step approach that consists of a positive mindset, physical activity, exercises, and healthy and nutritious recipes.

Healthy recipes ensure that although the calorie intake is greatly restricted, the body and its vital organs by extension receives all the important macro and micronutrients.

Feeding on unhealthy meals that consist of soft drinks, energy drinks, meals that are rich in simple starches, saturated fats and oils, and white foods is extremely detrimental to your body and may cause you to gain weight as opposed to losing it.

There are many foods that you could choose from to make a delicious meal that is still in line with the intermittent fasting diet. Below are some of the foods that constitute a healthy recipe:

Vegetables such as: broccoli, cauliflower, cucumber, tomatoes, beetroot, turnips, scallions, lettuce, bell peppers, spinach, and kales. These vegetables are best eaten raw or lightly steamed or boiled to avoid destroying important nutrients and vitamins.

Fruits such as: apples, bananas, grapes, strawberries, blueberries, lemon, lime, oranges, tangerines, pineapples, peaches, plums, gooseberries, and acai berries are also very important.

Nuts and seeds such as: almonds, walnuts, pistachios, pecan, macadamia, sunflower seeds, pumpkin seeds, and melon seeds.

Proteins from foods such as: chicken breast, lean cuts of pork and beef, tofu, eggs, beans, peas, black peas, and chickpeas.

Whole grains from foods such as: brown rice, oat, millet, quinoa, barley, and sorghum. These are cereals that are hardly refined.

Dairy products such as: buttermilk, full-fat milk, full-fat yogurt, cottage cheese, cheddar cheese, and ricotta cheese.

Healthy fats and oils from foods such as: olive oil, peanut butter, coconut oil, almond butter, avocados, and sunflower butter.

Healthy calorie-free beverages such as: unsweetened teas, coffees, homemade lemonade, coconut water, freshly made fruit juices, and most importantly, mineral water.

Some of the foods that you should avoid at all costs include: fatty cuts of beef and pork, flavored yogurt, cream cheese, white grains, vegetable oil, margarine, and mayonnaise.

9.2 Why do We Need Nutritious Recipes?

Nutritious recipes are meals that contain all the important macro and micronutrients that are required by the body. Each meal should have a healthy portion of these nutritious recipes, implying that the meal should not be too big, nor too small.

Nutritious recipes are often rich in fruits and vegetables. It is highly recommended that each recipe should contain at least three different types of fruits, and three different types of vegetables. This is because fruits and vegetables are very rich in both soluble and insoluble fibers. These fibers usually take a longer time to be digested, creating a feeling of fullness and reducing hunger pangs. In addition, insoluble fibers are important in preventing constipation. Fruits often contain plenty of vitamins and minerals which are important in improving the immunity of the body. Some fruits, such as the avocado, are rich in non-saturated fats which are extremely filling and satiating.

Furthermore, nutritious recipes often contain whole grains and foods. These are important because, unlike the white grains, they are not refined. This implies that they do not contain any synthetic vitamins and minerals.

The intermittent fasting diet is usually rich in proteins and fats and oils. To ensure that the diet is healthy and nutritious, nuts and seeds are used since they contain healthy fats and oils, which are important in keeping the body in a state of ketosis.

Proteins obtained from lean cuts of beef, pork, and bacon are also very important, since they contain healthy and nutritious protein, and most of the important amino acids. These proteins serve to strengthen your muscles and body organs, while keeping the glucose levels in the bloodstream low. In addition, proteins also reduce cravings and feelings of hunger, which are important in ensuring the success of an intermittent fasting diet.

Calorie-free beverages are also very important, as they provide you with the desired hydration to keep your body in perfect shape. Coffee is particularly considered to be very important, as it increases the metabolism of the body, leading to the increased burning of fat as a source of energy. In addition, coffee is important in reducing hunger pangs and cravings.

9.3 Some Healthy Recipes that you can Try During Intermittent Fasting

There are different recipes that you could try out at different times in the course of your feeding window or feeding day. These recipes will greatly depend on your dietary needs and physical activity at a particular point in time.

When breaking your fast, you should prepare meals that are rich in healthy fats but still low in calories. You should avoid binge eating or eating sugary foods when breaking your fast, as this has the potential to tire you out. Below are some of the recipes that you could try out when breaking your fast:

Recipe 1: Green Smoothie

Ingredients:

1 avocado

1 cup of coconut milk

1 handful of berries

1 cup of spinach or kale

1 cup of chia seeds

Method:

Place all the ingredients in a blender and blend until you achieve the desired consistency.

Recipe 2: Nut and Berry Parfait

Ingredients

6 crushed almonds

6 crushed walnuts

10 diced strawberries

1/3 cup blackberries

1/3 cup raspberries

½ tablespoon chia seeds

1 teaspoon cinnamon

1 teaspoon pure vanilla extract

½ cup heavy whipping cream

Method:

1. Place the whipping cream in a bowl and add the vanilla extract.
2. Use a hand mixer on medium and whip the whipped cream for about 2 to 3 minutes, or until stiff peaks form.
3. Stir the nuts and berries into the whipped cream.
4. Add in the chia seeds and sprinkle some cinnamon on the top.

Recipe 3: Grain-free Pancakes

Ingredients:

¼ cup of coconut flour

½ teaspoon of baking powder

1/4 teaspoon of salt

½ cup of whipped cream

7. eggs

1 teaspoon vanilla extract

½ tablespoon of organic honey

1 tablespoon butter

Ground cinnamon

Method:

1. Preheat the skillet over medium heat.
2. In a bowl, mix the eggs, vanilla and cream.
3. In a separate bowl, mix the coconut flour, baking soda and salt then gently stir in the wet ingredients into the dry ingredients.
4. Melt the butter in a skillet.
5. Pour about 2 to 3 tablespoons of butter into the skillet to form pancakes that are at least 10 cm in diameter.
6. Cook the pancakes for 2 -3 minutes on each side until golden brown.

7. Repeat the process until all the batter is over.

Below are some of the recipes that you could prepare for all other meals after you break your fast:

Recipe 4: Salmon and vegetables

Salmon is a type of fish that is rich in omega-3 oils, which are healthy fats that are nutritious.

Ingredients:

1 pound of salmon

2 tablespoons of lemon juice

2 tablespoons of ghee

4 cloves of garlic

Method:

1. Preheat the oven to 400°C

2. In a bowl, mix the lemon juice, ghee, and finely diced garlic.

3. Place the salmon in foil and pour the mixture above it.

4. Wrap the salmon in the foil and place it in a baking sheet.

5. Bake in the oven for 15 minutes or until the salmon is cooked. You could also roast your vegetables in a separate baking sheet or alongside the salmon.

Recipe 5: Grain-free Cauliflower Pizza

Ingredients:

1 pound of pizza florets

2 eggs, lightly beaten

1 teaspoon salt

1 teaspoon dried oregano

1 teaspoon garlic powder

Pizza toppings of your choice

Method:

1. Pre-heat the oven to 400°C.
2. Place the cauliflower in a food processor and pulse them until they are finely chopped, then transfer them to a large bowl.
3. In the bowl, add the eggs, salt, oregano and garlic powder and mix well.
4. Transfer the cauliflower mixture onto the

baking sheet and spread it to form the pizza crust.
5. Bake the crust for about 20 minutes, or until the crust is slightly golden.
6. Add your desired toppings then bake for 10 – 15 minutes.

Recipe 6: Chicken Drumsticks Wrapped in Bacon

Ingredients:

4 Chicken drumsticks

4 slices of bacon

1 ½ teaspoons of salt

1 teaspoon of ground pepper

Method:

1. Pre-heat the oven to 400°F. Line the baking sheet with aluminum foil.
2. Wrap a piece of bacon around the drumstick from the bottom to the top. Place the 4 drumsticks on the baking sheet and season with salt and pepper.
3. Bake for 45 minutes or until the bacon looks

golden.

Recipe 7: Strawberry and Kale Salad

Ingredients:

4 cups of kale

1 cup of walnuts

12 strawberries

1 tablespoon balsamic vinegar

4 tablespoons extra virgin oil

Salt and black pepper

Method:

1. In a large bowl, mix the kale, strawberries and walnuts.
2. Pour the vinegar and olive oil over the salad.
3. Season with salt and black pepper.

Recipe 8: Cinnamon Roll Fat Bombs

Ingredients:

1 teaspoon cinnamon

1 tablespoon coconut oil

2 tablespoons almond butter

½ cup coconut cream

Method:

1. Mix the cinnamon and the coconut cream.
2. Line a suitable baking pan with parchment paper and spread the cinnamon and coconut cream mixture.
3. Mix ½ a teaspoon of cinnamon with coconut oil and almond butter and spread over the first layer in the baking pan.
4. Freeze for about 10 minutes then cut into the desired squares or circular pieces.

Recipe 9: Homemade Chicken Strips

Ingredients:

1 pound of boneless chicken breasts trimmed to finger-like pieces

2 eggs

1 tablespoon of salt

1 teaspoon of freshly ground pepper

1 teaspoon of paprika

1 teaspoon of garlic

2 tablespoons of coconut oil

Hot sauce

Method:

1. Preheat the oven to 300°C and line the baking sheet with aluminum foil.
2. Wash the chicken fingers thoroughly and pat dry using some kitchen towels.
3. In a small bowl, combine the pork rinds, salt, pepper, paprika and garlic. Pour the mixture into a sealable bag.
4. In a larger bowl, beat the eggs and dip each fish finger into the egg wash to coat.
5. Add the chicken breasts that are coated with the egg into the sealable bag with the spice mixture.
6. Seal the bag to allow the mixture to coat the chicken.
7. Place the chicken strips on the baking sheet and place them in the oven. Allow to bake for about 10 – 15 minutes.
8. Flip the chicken over and allow it to cook for another 10 – 15 minutes until golden brown

in color. Remove the chicken from the oven and allow it to cool for 5 minutes before serving.

9. Serve with some hot sauce on the side.

Recipe 10: Chicken Wings

Ingredients:

2 pounds chicken wings

1 tablespoon of salt

1 teaspoon of paprika

1 teaspoon of freshly ground black pepper

1 tablespoon of baking powder

1 teaspoon of garlic

2 tablespoons of coconut oil

2 tablespoons of hot sauce

Method:

1. Wash the chicken wings and pat dry.
2. In a small bowl, combine the salt, pepper, baking powder, paprika, and garlic.
3. Place the wings in a sealable plastic bag and

add the spice mixture.
4. Seal and shake the bag to coat the wings.
5. Preheat a skillet over medium heat and melt the coconut oil in the warm pan.
6. Place the wings in the skillet and cover.
7. Cook for 10 to 12 minutes.
8. Flip the wings and cook for another 10 to 12 minutes, until golden brown.
9. Remove the wings from the heat and let cool for 5 minutes.
10. Coat the wings with hot sauce, if desired.

Recipe 11: Chicken Stuffed Bell-peppers

Ingredients:

1 tablespoon of butter

1 clove garlic, minced

1 small onion, diced

1 teaspoon of paprika

1 teaspoon of salt

½ teaspoon of freshly ground black pepper

1 teaspoon of chili powder

1 cup grape tomatoes, halved

1-pound ground chicken

3 beaten eggs

4 large bell peppers, halved

Instructions:

1. Preheat the oven to 350°F. Line a baking sheet with parchment paper.
2. Melt the butter in a skillet over medium heat. Add the garlic, onion, salt, pepper, paprika, and chili powder, then sauté for 5 to 7 minutes.
3. Add the tomatoes and sauté for another 5 to 7 minutes.
4. Add the ground chicken and cook until golden brown, about 15 minutes, stirring occasionally.
5. Transfer the cooked meat mixture to a medium-sized bowl and slowly mix in the eggs.
6. Lay each bell pepper half cut side up on the prepared baking sheet.
7. Pour the meat and egg mixture into the bell peppers.

8. Place the stuffed peppers in the oven and bake for 60 minutes, until the peppers soften slightly.

Recipe 12: Simple Homemade bacon

Ingredients:

2 pounds pork belly

⅔ cup salt

2 tablespoons of freshly ground black pepper

Any dried herbs and spices

Method:

1. Remove the skin from the pork belly with a very sharp knife. As you remove it, try to keep the skin intact.
2. Rinse the pork belly and pat dry with a kitchen towel.
3. In a small bowl, mix together the salt, pepper, and any dried herbs and spices.
4. Rub the mixture on both sides of the pork belly.
5. Place the pork belly inside a sealed airtight container and store in the refrigerator for 5

to 7 days. The flavor becomes stronger the longer you cure it.
6. Flip the pork belly over every day. (Make sure you wash your hands thoroughly before touching the pork belly.)
7. After 5 to 7 days, remove the pork belly from the refrigerator and rinse off the salt, pepper, and any other herbs and spices. Pat dry.
8. Preheat the oven to 200°F (90°C).
9. Place a roasting rack in a roasting pan. Place the pork belly fat side up on the rack.
10. Bake until the meat reaches an internal temperature of 150°F. This usually takes about an hour and a half to two hours.
11. Remove the pork belly from the oven and let it cool for 30 minutes.
12. Wrap the meat in parchment paper and store in the refrigerator overnight or for 12 hours.

Recipe 13: Grass-Fed Burgers

Ingredients:

½ teaspoon of garlic powder

½ teaspoon of cumin powder

½ pound of ground grass-fed beef liver

½ pound of ground grass-fed beef

Sea salt and pepper to taste

Desired cooking oil

Method:

1. Mix together all ingredients in a bowl and form patties of your desired size.
2. Heat cooking oil over a skillet on medium-high heat.
3. Cook burgers in skillet until desired.
4. Store in a container in the fridge and use within 4 days.

Your Quick Start Action Step:
Once you begin your intermittent fasting diet, you should always schedule time to plan your meals. This, of course, involves creating time to visit the local market to stock up your kitchen cabinets and refrigerator.

This section provides you with guidance on some of the foods that you could include in your meal plan, and those that are strictly forbidden. Hence, this will give you some guidance to help you in meal planning. As a disclaimer, you must note that the foods are not limited to those listed in this section.

Once you begin your intermittent fasting diet, you could choose a recipe from the above list of recipes. Recipes 1 – 3 are mainly prepared when you want to break your fast. The rest of the recipes can be prepared for other times of the day.

The recipes for the intermittent fasting diet are widely available across the internet and print media. As such, do not feel limited to the ones that we have listed in this section. You can always try out different recipes and stick to specific ones, depending on the recipes that you like best.

Chapter 10: Mistakes to Avoid and Who Should Not Fast

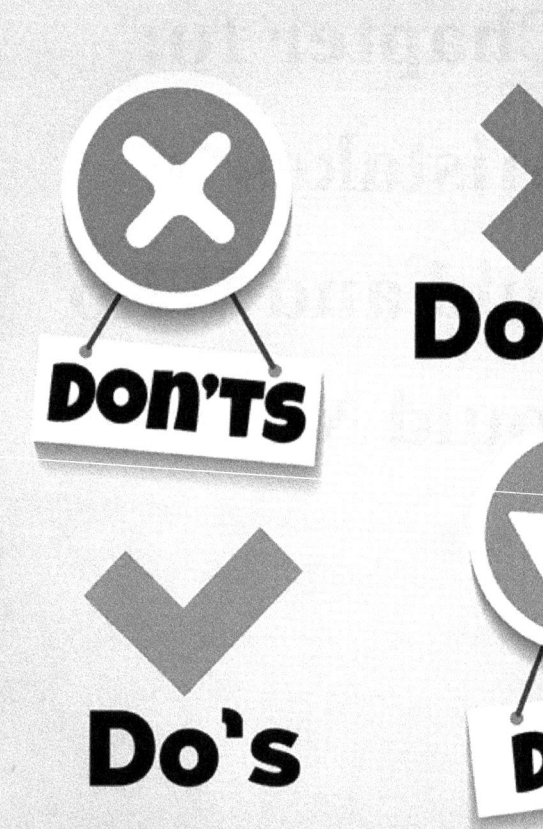

Chapter 10: Mistakes to Avoid and Who Should Not Fast

10.1 Brief Introduction

Many people find intermittent fasting to be an extreme measure and opt for other methods to shed off some of the extra pounds that they want to lose. However, the people who have tried this method can attest to its success in weight loss, and some of the additional benefits that come with it. The method is especially preferred because it ensures that you do not gain the pounds that you have successfully shed off, keeping you healthy lean and fit.

The proponents of this method do however agree that it is difficult, and it is not meant for everyone. This method of weight loss calls for a lot of personal discipline, commitment, and resilience. Throughout the whole process, your willpower will be tested countless times in ways that you cannot imagine or believe to have been possible.

Many people who get on the intermittent fasting

diet attest to the fact that getting over the hunger pangs and the food cravings will take a lot of personal discipline and motivation. Most of the time, people are advised to ignore the discomfort that comes with the hunger and instead focus on the goal that they intend to achieve.

However, the hardest part about the whole process is getting over the habit of having three meals each day. Habits are very dangerous because they become ingrained in us and form part of our personality. As such, changing the habit of having three meals a day becomes very difficult.

In addition, the feeling of hunger is controlled by the hormone known as ghrelin. The natural circadian rhythm, which controls the release of the ghrelin hormone, does not follow the eat/fast routine of the intermittent fasting diet. As such, you may find that the moments in which the quantity of the ghrelin hormone is high coincide with your fasting window.

However, here's a piece of encouragement: the

beginning is the hardest part, it gets better! All you will need to do is to maintain a positive mindset and surround yourself with positive people, preferably those who share the same goals as you. In no time at all, you will find yourself able to fast for longer hours of time without experiencing any feelings of hunger or cravings.

10.2 A List of People Who Should Not Fast

Based on the extreme nature of the intermittent fasting diet, it is not suitable for everyone. If you have read this book and are attracted to the potential benefits that this diet has in relation to your health and general wellbeing, then you are advised to seek the advice of a medical practitioner or nutritionist.

When you begin the fasting process, you will need to carefully monitor your body for any signs of weakness, dizziness, light-headedness, moodiness, or even constipation. If you observe these symptoms, you are advised to stop the fasting diet and consult the experts on the way forward. The suffering and discomfort that you will experience is simply not worth it.

Pregnant and lactating women are strongly advised against intermittent fasting. This is because they have additional energy needs for the growing fetus and, in the case of lactating women, for the growing baby who depends on breast milk for nourishment. Such women are advised to try out the diet once they have given birth and have breastfed for at least 6 months.

People who have a history of eating disorders are also strongly advised against trying out the intermittent fasting diet. This is because such people already have a history of abnormal and disturbed eating habits, which include anorexia and bulimia nervosa. Fasting may create additional problems for you which may make your situation worse than it already was.

If you are chronically stressed, then it probably is not a good idea for you to create additional stress for your body. The elevated heart rate, high blood pressure, and high levels of stress hormones from chronic stress are already taking a toll on your body. Fasting periods are only going to make your body more stressed and you may not achieve your intended goals.

People who have both type 1 and type 2 diabetes are generally advised against intermittent fasting. In some situations, fasting has led to an increase in blood pressure, and the cholesterol levels in the body, while in other situations, it has reduced the insulin levels and the blood pressure levels. As such, if you are interested in intermittent fasting, you are advised to seek the advice of your doctor.

Anyone who does not get the recommended eight hours of sleep is highly advised to avoid fasting. Inadequate sleep already stresses the body and affects your health. Fasting is likely to make your body deteriorate further. As such, you are more likely to experience feelings of weakness and lightheadedness.

If your lifestyle does not fit into the intermittent fasting process, you should avoid forcing yourself to adopt it. This is because essentially, it is the intermittent diet that is supposed to fit into your life and not the other way around.

Lastly, you should not get on the intermittent fasting diet if you are not interested and most of all passionate about it. Being an extremely demanding process, you will only set yourself up for failure and misery.

10.3 Mistakes to Avoid When Fasting

If you are passionate about intermittent fasting as a tool to lose weight and you convince yourself to give it a try, then there are many pitfalls that you will need to avoid if you are going to be successful. Below are some of the most common mistakes when it comes to intermittent fasting:

1. Inasmuch as intermittent fasting is hard, many people come in with this preconceived notion and end up throwing in the towel too soon. The truth of the matter is that the beginning is the hardest part, it gets better! All you will need to do is to maintain a positive mindset and surround yourself with positive people, preferably those who share

the same goals as you. In no time at all, you will find yourself able to fast for longer hours of time without experiencing any feelings of hunger or cravings.
2. On the flip side of the coin, many other people approach the diet with a can-do mentality and end up jumping in way too fast. The problem with this is that such people will set very unrealistic goals, which will end up discouraging them altogether. As such, beginners are advised to start with small but attainable goals which will keep them motivated.
3. Beginners who are just trying out the intermittent fasting process will often put their lives on hold and exclusively focus on fasting to lose weight. This is a mistake, as you will notice the hunger that you are feeling and get tempted to grab a meal during your fasting period. Essentially, you should keep yourself busy to take your mind off your stomach until it is time to break your fast.
4. While there are many ways in which you

could go about the intermittent fasting diet, many people often lack guidance, and end up choosing a wrong plan which will only serve to stress you out and make you miserable. As I have repeated several times, the intermittent diet is supposed to fit into your lifestyle and not the other way around. This is the only way in which the habit will stick.

5. Since you will not get many opportunities to eat, both the quantity and quality of the food that you eat will be very important in determining the success of your fast. Due to the extreme nature of the fast, people often tend to feed on anything they come across without considering its nutritional content, a habit that could easily result in weight gain. As a general rule of thumb, your food should contain healthy portions of all the macronutrients. Starches and simple sugars should however be minimized in order to keep the body in a state of ketosis.

6. People often forget to remain hydrated, most especially during the fasting window. People

forget that it is acceptable to have beverages such as mineral water, unsweetened teas, and coffees while fasting. As a matter of fact, these drinks are extremely important as they help to keep hunger at bay and reduce the cravings.

7. When the time to break the fast comes, many people binge eat and feast to make up for the hunger that they experienced during the fasting window. This is a mistake because binge eating will cause your blood sugar levels to sharply increase. Once you resume your fast, the blood sugar levels will also sharply decrease. The fluctuations in the blood sugar levels will lead to moodiness, weakness, and dizziness, which will make it harder to stick to the diet. It is recommended that you should break your fast on a meal that contains 300 – 400 calories.

8. Some people fail to eat enough during the feeding window. Due to lack of knowledge and the fear that they will undo the benefits that they have gained from the fast, many people will eat less than the required

amounts. As such, the body will kick into starvation mode by cannibalizing your muscle mass and slowing down your metabolism. This will make it even more difficult to lose weight.

9. Some people may decide to take the whole intermittent fasting process too far, making it difficult to stick to it. Essentially, methods such as the 16/8 method, eat-stop-eat method, and 5:2 method are meant for beginners as you will only need to fast for relatively shorter periods of time. People who decide to begin with the 4:3 method or the 3:3 method often take it too far and end up giving up.

10. Due to all the rage that is associated with intermittent fasting, many people often try out the method hoping to lose weight quickly and gain the associated benefits. However, some people end up forcing the process to work so much so that they forget that weight loss is a three-part process that involves a positive mindset and physical activity, in addition to the diet. Hence, people forget

that there are many other ways of losing weight that do not necessarily involve fasting.

11. The constant, and to some extent, obsessive fear of the feeling of hunger is yet another mistake that people make. People often fear that the body will waste away, and they will die even before the fasting window comes to an end. As such, they respond to the slightest form of hunger by breaking the fast and eventually do not gain anything from the fasting process. Instead, people should avoid any feelings of hunger and rely on the body to produce ketones as an alternative source of fuel.

Your Quick Start Action Step:

Essentially, anyone can take part in intermittent fasting, apart from the people that have been mentioned in the list above. If you are lucky enough to be able to take part in the diet, I would advise you learn from the mistakes of others, as it is only a fool who insists on making their own mistakes.

You are therefore advised to take into consideration some of the common mistakes that have been highlighted and avoid these pitfalls.

Chapter 11: When You Are Not Seeing Results

Chapter 11: When You Are Not Seeing Results

11.1 Expect That Not All the Results Will Happen

Intermittent fasting is widely famed for all the benefits that it is believed to offer the human body. Some of these benefits include: weight loss, reduced inflammation, improved mental functionality, decreased blood sugar levels, increased insulin sensitivity, and the retarded growth of tumors.

However, human bodies are inherently different, and each body reacts differently to the intermittent fasting process. Some people who fast for extended durations of time may reap all these benefits, some people may reap only a few of these benefits, and others will reap none at all.

If you end up reaping all the benefits, then congratulations to you! If you only reap some of the benefits or even none at all, take courage. Take this as an opportunity to go back to the drawing board to analyze some of the mistakes that you may have made that could have prevented you from reaping these benefits. In addition, make sure to consult a medical practitioner or nutritionist to advise you on the way forward.

One of the main reasons why the fasting process may have failed is that you did not focus on the foods that you were consuming. It could be that you focused on consuming all the wrong foods and did not pay attention to the foods that are required for the intermittent fasting process. Consuming foods that are rich in starches and simple sugars might have caused you to gain weight as opposed to losing it.

Alternatively, it could be that you either consumed too much food or too little food whenever you broke your fast. Consuming little food might have caused your body's metabolism to slow down resulting in an inability to break down fats. Binge eating, otherwise known as feasting, may have increased the calories that you consumed, leading to weight gain as opposed to loss.

Alternatively, you could have chosen a method that could not work for your lifestyle, and that made it extremely difficult for you to follow through with it. You might also have been too aggressive in your approach towards intermittent fasting which may have made it impossible for you to achieve your goals.

In addition, you may find that you were not motivated or enthusiastic about intermittent fasting which greatly affected your morale, making it impossible to achieve some of the goals that you were hoping to. This could have occurred if you were simply following the crowd. On the other hand, you may have done everything perfectly but still failed to achieve the results that you were hoping for. If this is the case, intermittent fasting is probably not suitable for you. You may want to consider other methods of weight loss which are equally as effective and beneficial to your health and general wellbeing.

You must also be aware that some of these results may take longer to manifest in your body compared to other people. This is because we are all genetically different and some of our biological processes may differ greatly from one person to the next. This should not be a cause for alarm but, instead, a call for you to exercise patience and constancy in the pursuit of your goal.

11.2 Importance of Being Aware of This

Being aware that some of the results may take time to manifest is very important, as it will keep you optimistic and enthusiastic about the intermittent fasting process. It will keep you from giving up and probably motivate you to push your boundaries even further to test your limits.

In addition, knowledge that it is not all the results that will manifest on everyone is important as it will keep you from bad-mouthing the entire fasting process and will allow other people to explore the method without feeling discouraged by your results. In some situations, being aware of this will place you in a better position to advise and motivate others, especially beginners.

11.3 What to Do When the Results Do Not Happen

1. The first thing that you should do if you do not get the results that you intended is to get back to the drawing board and carefully analyze all the steps that you took, being careful to identify any mistakes that you could have made in the process. To make the examination thorough, you could seek the help of a friend to help you to go through the entire process.

2. Once this is done, you should list down all the mistakes that you made and conduct extensive and in-depth research on the correct way to go about these processes. As always, knowledge is power, and the process of learning never stops!

3. You could also seek the advice of your doctor, a medical practitioner, or a nutritionist to provide you with useful insights as to why the process did not work. It could be that you are suffering from a pre-existent condition which made it difficult to

follow through with the fasting process, which prevented some of results from happening.

4. If you still believe in intermittent fasting as the key to weight loss, you could join a group of people who are fasting for the same purpose. This will ensure that you have people that you can compare notes with, and who can motivate you to hit your goals whenever you get side-tracked. Alternatively, you could simply request a family member or a friend to become your accountability partner.

5. When the results do not happen because of a poor diet, you could work on improving your fasting diet. First, you could go shopping at your local grocery store or supermarket to source all the ingredients that you will need to prepare healthy and nutritious meals. The foods should have healthy portions of all the major nutrients. Second, take time off your busy schedule to plan for the meals that you will have during each feeding window. Proper meal planning will ensure that you

neither under-feed, nor over-feed whenever you break your fast.

6. If you failed to achieve your results due to low commitment and motivation, find a way to keep yourself constantly motivated to achieve your goals. This could be through maintaining a spreadsheet that will track all your progress.
7. If you fail to achieve one of your small goals, find a way to pick yourself up and get back on the horse. You must always remember to be kind to yourself. Whenever you achieve, and possibly even surpass your goals, always find a way to pat yourself on the back, either by giving yourself a gift or rewarding yourself with a cheat day to enjoy some of your favorite meals.
8. You could also focus on setting goals that are less ambitious and more realistic. For starters, you should select a fasting method that caters for shorter fasting windows and longer feeding windows. This is because adjusting from your normal life to the fasting diet will ordinarily require a huge

paradigm shift, and extreme discipline. This will probably make it more possible to achieve your goals.

9. Nonetheless, it is important to never force the process on yourself or on your life. If it does not flow naturally, or fit into your lifestyle, then it is probably time that you admitted this to yourself and found alternative ways to lose the weight, and to gain the additional benefits that come with intermittent fasting. The good news is that there are plenty of dietary plans which are available out there, and still as effective. Physical activity and exercises are also recommended. For some of the added benefits, you could use various supplements which will boost your health in the process.

Your Quick Start Action Step:
As such, whenever you fail to achieve the results you had hoped for, you will need to remember that it is not the end of the world, and that there are many more ways that you could use to achieve your goals.

Refer to the above steps which will guide you on some of the areas that you can improve on, and if not, other recommended ways of shedding off the extra pounds, and enjoying the results of the fasting diet without necessarily being on one.

Bearing this in mind, you must pick yourself up, dust yourself off, put on a brave face, and go forth to correct some of the mistakes that you might have made. Again, you must never forget that fasting is indeed a lifestyle and not merely a one-time thing. This will help you to realize that most of the results will not be achieved in the blink of an eye, nor will they be achieved in a couple of weeks, or months. You will need to persistently and diligently put in the effort, while setting your sights on the bigger goal that you aim to achieve.

You will also need to remember that the intermittent fasting diet will require your time in meal planning and meal preparation. Hence, always make sure to schedule time in the course of your busy day to do these activities which are likely to make all the difference.

Chapter 12: Living the Healthy, Guilt-Free Lifestyle

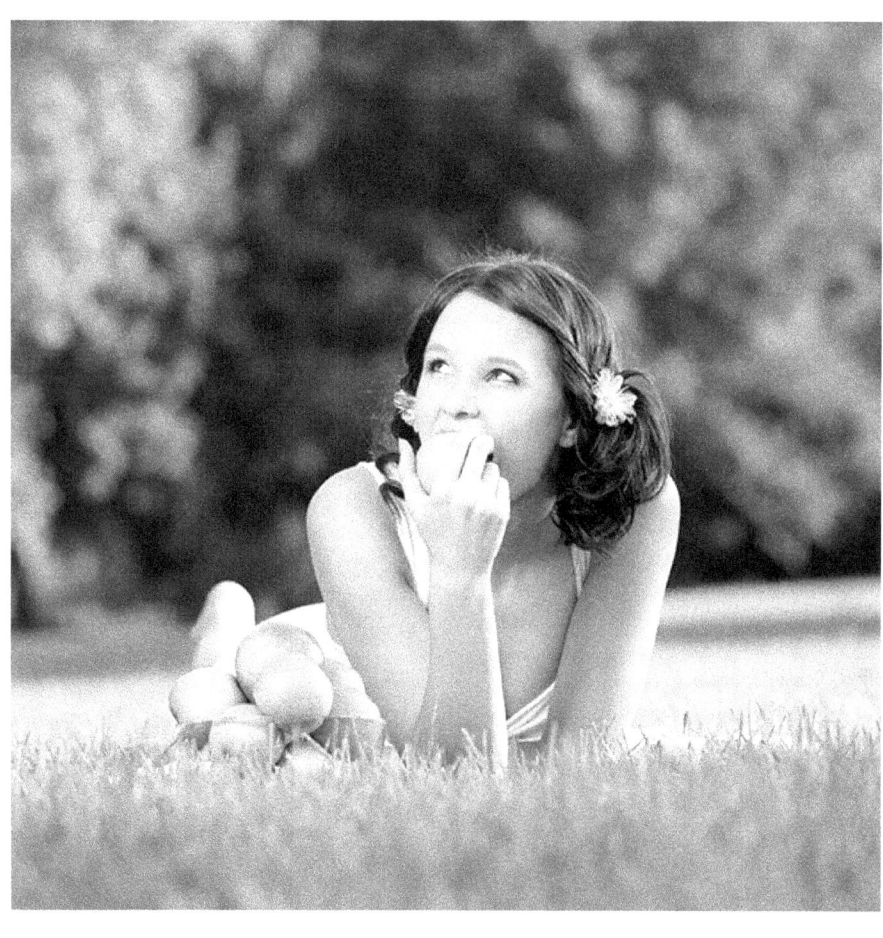

Chapter 12: Living the Healthy, Guilt-Free Lifestyle

12.1 Intermittent Fasting as a Lifestyle

By now, you must have realized that despite the hype and the craze that is associated with the intermittent fasting diet, one important fact that many people fail to consider is that fasting is not merely a dietary plan, or a one-hit-wonder. It is a lifestyle, a way of life.

Intermittent fasting uses a holistic way in approaching the problem of weight loss. It is a three-part process that encompasses your mindset, the fitness and exercise levels, and most of all, your dietary plan, which is where the intermittent fasting diet comes in.

As such, the benefits of this diet are not merely weight loss, but include increasing insulin sensitivity, reducing blood sugar levels, reducing inflammations in the body, longevity and slow aging, increased metabolism, and the retarded growth of cancer cells.

Despite being one of the fastest and most effective methods of losing weight, optimal results will only be expected when you combine the diet with healthy nutrition and a healthy lifestyle.

The foods that you consume should be rich in important minerals, vitamins, and other nutrients which are important in ensuring proper bodily functions. Junk foods, foods that are rich in starch and simple sugars, carbonated drinks, white refined foods, and fatty cuts of meat are generally considered unhealthy and should not be consumed while on the intermittent fasting diet.

Physical exercise and workouts are also highly recommended, despite the low energy levels that are experienced while fasting. These exercises are mainly recommended for individuals who have been on the diet for a while and are comfortable in fasting. The exercise should not be intensive but should stretch the bodily organs and make sure that the muscles are well toned. This will prevent saggy skin after the weight loss.

The mindset is also an important aspect of the intermittent fasting process. In general, one's mindset should be very positive and optimistic when going into this diet. A few weeks or months into the diet, you will learn the important skills of resilience and personal discipline, which will serve to strengthen your willpower and contribute to making you a better person.

12.2 Why Intermittent Fasting is Worth it in the End

While it is unanimously agreed upon that intermittent fasting is a daunting and difficult task, proponents of the method still believe that it is one of the most effective weight loss programs, as it often improves on different aspects of your general lifestyle and wellbeing. Once you achieve some of these goals or results, the trouble that you went through while fasting becomes insignificant.

Below are some of the reasons why intermittent fasting is worth it:

Unlike most other dietary plans and fasting methods, none guarantees people that they will not regain the weight that they have lost. These methods only cater for the weight loss part and leave the maintenance of the new weight to you. Seeing as many people fail to maintain their new weight on their own, the intermittent fasting diet tops the list.

Intermittent fasting is unique as it results in an extended lifespan. Intermittent fasting diets are believed to alter the mitochondrial networks inside the energy producing cells, increasing lifespan, and promoting good health.

The intermittent fasting diet has also been proven to have benefits for patients suffering from type 2 diabetes. As a result of the decreased insulin levels in the bloodstream, the cells become more sensitive to any insulin released into the bloodstream. As such, it does not accumulate within the blood. This then leads to an improvement in insulin sensitivity.

The growth of carcinogenic tumors is also retarded. Periodic fasting leads to a decrease in the growth of cancerous tumors and increased sensitivity to chemotherapy. When cancerous cells are exposed to environments that contain lower glucose levels, proliferation and cell death quickly follow, a process known as cell starvation.

Through intermittent fasting, we have a significant decrease in inflammation in the body. Inflammation is a common symptom of all chronic diseases that we face today. It is known to occur whenever the body is trying to heal itself. However, whenever inflammation occurs for too long, it is associated with some negative effects.

Improved brain functionality and cognitive functions also comes up when the body uses ketones as sources of energy, as opposed to the conventional glucose.

12.3 Steps on How to Maintain a Healthy Lifestyle

1. One should focus on eating healthy meals and drinking calorie-free drinks such as water, unsweetened teas, and coffee. Feeding on unhealthy meals that consist of soft drinks, energy drinks, meals that are rich in simple starches, saturated fats and

oils, and white foods is extremely detrimental to your body.

2. Boost your intake of fruits and vegetables. Fruits and vegetables are an important constituent of a healthy diet. They are rich in nutrients, minerals and phytonutrients, which boost the individual's immunity and help to fight disease-causing organisms.

3. Consume foods that are rich in fibers. Fibers often absorb water when in the gut. This causes them to become soft and bulky. This reduces constipation by making the bowel movements easier.

4. Cut down on processed foods. These foods are often stripped of important nutrients and replaced with synthetic nutrients. Some of them even contain preservatives, which may be harmful to your health. Opt for organic foods as opposed to processed foods.

5. Choose white meats over red meats. Red meats have been linked to increased risk of colon cancer, and increased cholesterol levels. White meats on the other hand are

very nutritious. Fish for example is rich in omega-3 oils and vitamin D.

6. Keep your body physically fit and well-toned by visiting the gym, taking long walks, participating in yoga, or carrying out simple exercises from the comfort of your own home. Depending on your age, medical factors, ethnicity, and other factors, you could choose between low, moderate, and high-intensity exercises.
7. Maintain a healthy weight, and by extension, a healthy Body Mass Index (BMI). A healthy Body Mass Index is found anywhere between 18.5 and 24.9.
8. Avoid smoking and restrict your alcohol intake as much as possible. Smoking is generally unhealthy, as it leads to many other diseases and complications. As such, it should be avoided at all costs.
9. Avoid eating very heavy meals at a go. Instead, focus on consuming light meals at frequent intervals. This will keep your blood sugar levels in check and prevent the feelings

of drowsiness and moodiness that often come with unstable levels of blood sugar.

10. Replace saturated fats with unsaturated fats. Saturated fats have the potential of increasing your cholesterol levels. This is harmful to your health and could result in cardiovascular disease and other heart diseases.

11. Keep your body hydrated by consuming plenty of mineral water, freshly squeezed juices, and calorie-free drinks. Essentially, you should drink at least eight glasses of water each day. This will keep your skin supple and your body organs functional.

12. Reduce your intake of salts and sugar. Salt has the potential of increasing your blood pressure, as well as the risk of cardiovascular diseases, and other heart diseases. When shopping, try to identify foods that are low in sodium. In addition, avoid adding salt at the dinner table. Although sugar is sweet and attractive, it should only be enjoyed in moderation as it could lead to high blood pressure.

13. Meet your daily sleep requirements. Sleep is an important factor that is often overlooked. Sleep gives your body rest by helping your muscles to recover. In addition, it keeps you looking younger and prevents you from aging! You should always aim for 6 – 7 hours of sleep every night.
14. Take time off your busy schedule to meditate. This will quieten down your body and soul and allow them to be one. This is especially important for concentration.

Your Quick Start Action Step:

Living a healthy lifestyle is a process that not only involves your dietary intake, but also your physical activity levels and your ability to stick to the process.

To live a healthy lifestyle, you should consider following the above-mentioned steps. The most important part about following these steps is having a can-do-mentality and remaining committed throughout the process. This could be achieved by surrounding yourself with like-minded people who will push you towards a healthy lifestyle.

In as much as the list above provides a conclusive list of some of the steps that you could take to live a healthy lifestyle, you must realize that it is not exclusive and there are many other steps that you could take to maintain a healthy lifestyle.

Bonus Chapter: Benefits with Ketogenic Diet

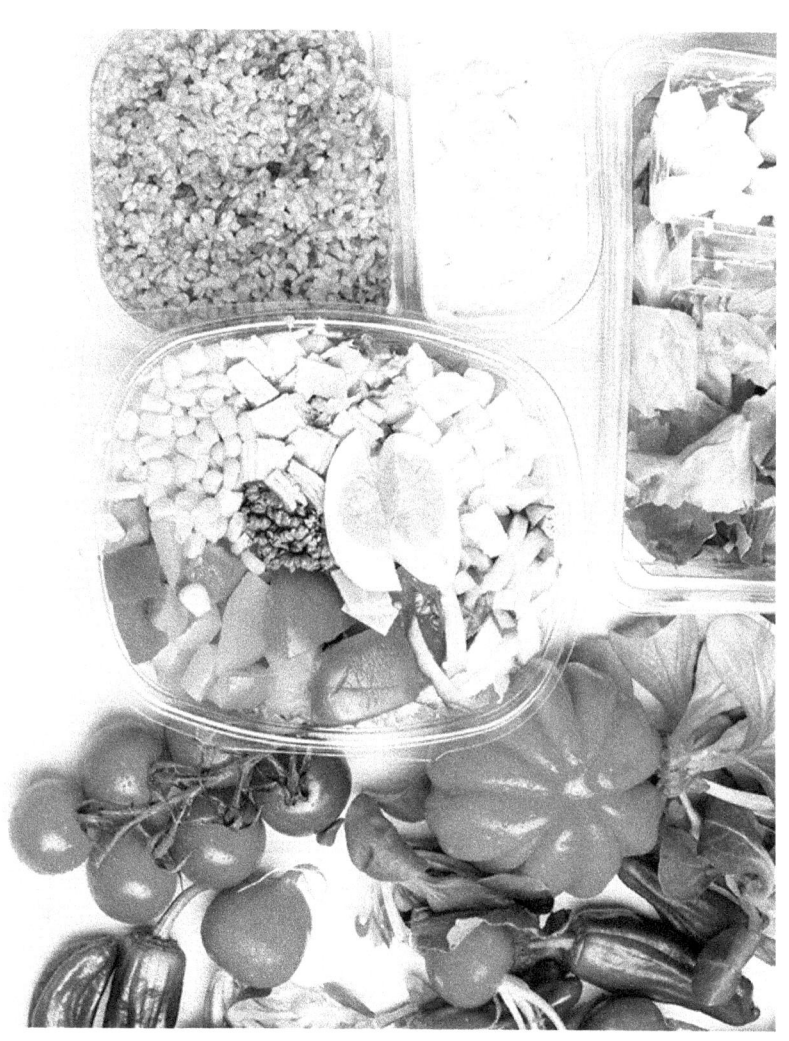

Bonus Chapter: Benefits with Ketogenic Diet

12.1 Background Information on the Ketogenic Diet

You've probably heard of the phrase 'keto diet' used amongst fitness experts and other individuals looking to hit their fitness goals. The ketogenic diet, often shortened to the keto diet, has become one of the most popular ways to shed off a few extra kilos. Despite its recent hype, the diet has been used by medical experts for more than one hundred years. It was initially popularized in the early 1920s and 1930s as a dietary therapy for epileptic patients. Today, the diet has proven benefits for weight loss, and the general health and performance of epileptic and diabetic patients.

The ketogenic diet has its roots in the ancient practice of fasting, and other dietary regimes that were used as treatment for epilepsy. These ancient practices were used from as early as 500 B.C., in the days of the ancient Greeks. These treatments included the excess or limitation of some animal, plant, or mineral substances. In the early 1920s, modern physicians began to mimic the biochemical effects of fasting and starvation to treat epilepsy. A pair of French physicians, were the first to record the use of starvation as a treatment for epilepsy. The pair treated 20 children and adults and reported that the seizures were less during the treatment period. For the next two decades, physicians and medical doctors conducted widespread research and tests on this method of treatment, during which the method was widely used. The use of the diet however declined in the late 1930s after the discovery of anti-convulsant drugs.

In the 1970s, a very low carbohydrate diet for weight loss was popularized by Dr. Atkins in his paper. The diet began with a two-week ketogenic phase that allowed for zero intake of carbohydrates. This was followed by a gradual addition of carbohydrates that ensured that the body kept burning its fat as fuel. Hence, individuals would continue to lose without hunger. In the long-term, individuals were to engage in meals containing 60% fats, 30% protein, and 10% carbohydrates. However, the followers of Atkin's diet were at a risk of having cancer, constipation, and malnutrition, amongst other health risks. Today, many years later, many fad diets still incorporate the same approach to weight loss.

That said, what then is a ketogenic diet? The ketogenic diet is a high-fat, low-carb, and moderate-protein meal plan. It entails eating foods that are rich in fats and reducing the intake of carbohydrates. It typically includes foods such as: meat, eggs, cheese, milk, processed meat, nuts, butter, oils, and seeds.

In the presence of carbohydrates, the body normally converts carbohydrates into glucose, which is then transported throughout the body to provide energy to perform different bodily functions. However, in the absence of carbohydrates, the liver breaks down fats into fatty acids and ketone bodies. The ketone bodies are then passed into the bloodstream, replacing glucose as a source of energy. As such, the body burns fats rather than carbohydrates to produce energy, a state known as ketosis. Generally, with a carbohydrate intake of less than 20 to 50 grams per day, the body takes about two to four days to shift from using circulating glucose to breaking down stored fats for energy.

While on a ketogenic diet, the body switches from glucose to ketones as the primary source of fuel supply. The body then increases the burning of fat, leading to a significant decrease in insulin levels in the bloodstream. This then becomes important to individuals who are trying to lose weight, for it makes it easier for the body to access and burn off fat reserves without the feeling of hunger or a decrease in the supply of energy, as is common with people who are fasting. However, it is argued that a ketogenic diet is more of a short-term diet that a long-term lifestyle. This is because of the social restrictions that the diet imposes on an individual. Scientific research also indicates that weight loss results after being on a ketogenic diet for 12 months are the same as those of individuals on a healthy diet.

In addition to people who are trying to lose weight, the ketogenic diet is also important to people with type 2 diabetes. Ketogenic diets assist the body in controlling blood sugar levels by reducing the amount of glucose in the bloodstream. This is known as glycemic control. As a result, the diet reduces the amount of insulin medication that a patient is required to take. However, keeping in mind that ketogenic diets include a high intake of fats, if the fats are saturated or of poor quality, then this may put a patient at a risk for cardiovascular diseases. A fat saturated diet leads to an increase in harmful cholesterol, placing one at a risk of heart problems. As such, people with type 2 diabetes are required to consult with their doctors before getting on a ketogenic diet.

There is also solid evidence dating back to more than one hundred years that seems to point out that, indeed, a ketogenic diet does reduce epileptic seizures especially in children. Because of these neuroprotective effects, physicians and medical doctors have been investigating any possible benefits for other brain disorders such as autism, Alzheimer's, and even Parkinson's disease. Hence, the ketogenic diet has proven to be important to people suffering from epilepsy.

The ketogenic diet, as we have seen, is a very important alternative in treating diabetes and epilepsy as well as in weight loss. However, the diet could become unhealthy if individuals partake in too much red meat, fatty foods, processed foods, and salty foods. These foods have the potential to complicate the situation further by introducing other complications such as heart problems. However, a balanced and unprocessed ketogenic diet that is rich in lean meats, fish, nuts, olive oils, seeds, whole grains, fruits, and vegetables is more likely to lead to a long and happy life.

The ketogenic diet is often used interchangeably with the intermittent fasting diet. This is because the condition of being overweight, and by extension, obesity, is mainly caused by the insulin hormone in the bloodstream. Being a fat storage hormone, whenever you consume more calories than your body needs, the insulin levels will rise and will stimulate the body to store the excess glucose as fat reserves within the body, leading to weight gain.

Hence, the ketogenic diet and the intermittent fasting diet are mainly based on the principle of reducing the insulin levels in the bloodstream to prevent the accumulation of fat deposits. Both diets also boost the ketone levels in the bloodstream and make the body burn more fats. When used simultaneously, these two methods are guaranteed to boost your weight loss and to improve your health and general wellbeing.

While it is true that you can use each of these methods independently, you will realize that it is more practical to use them simultaneously rather than independently. This is because intermittent fasting while on a ketogenic diet gives a significant boost to your weight loss journey, and vice versa is consequently true.

12.2 The Link between Intermittent Fasting and the Keto Diet

Having noted that intermittent fasting and the ketogenic diet affect the body in the same way, we will need to explore the link between these two methods of weight loss to understand just why it is that they work together so well.

Recall that the ketogenic diet is a high-fat, low-carb, and moderate-protein meal plan that results in a state of ketosis. By consuming fewer carbohydrates, there is less glucose, and by extension, less insulin in the bloodstream. The body then burns down its fat reserves to release energy in the form of ketones. Increased fat loss then results in weight loss.

Hence, keto dieters will have low blood sugar and low insulin levels. They will also be fully into the fat-burning mode, ketosis. The elevated ketones in the bloodstream and the satiating effects of the ketogenic diet will result in a reduced appetite, less hunger pangs, and cravings. These effects will especially be beneficial to people who are practicing intermittent fasting.

The ketogenic diet is believed to result in hunger suppression, which is important to people practicing intermittent fasting. The elevated ketones in the body suppress the production of the ghrelin hormone. The ghrelin hormone is based on the natural circadian rhythm and is responsible for hunger. Low levels of ghrelin reduce the feeling of hunger, even when you do not have any food in your system. As such, you can go for longer without eating anything and fasting becomes easier.

As mentioned earlier, the ketogenic diet is rich in fats and oils. Fats and oils do not spike your blood sugar levels. Instead, they stabilize the sugar levels. As such, pairing a ketogenic diet with intermittent fasting will result in stable and low blood sugar levels. This will eliminate any fatigue, mood swings, and cravings that may be associated with high-carb fasting. As such, combining the two methods could be especially useful to people suffering from type 2 diabetes.

In addition, high-carb diets will cause your blood sugar levels to rise whenever you break your fast, and to drop significantly during your fasting window. Unstable blood sugar levels will negatively impact the intermittent fasting process as they will result in sleepiness, low energy, mood swings, and intense cravings. If this keeps happening, intermittent fasting becomes very difficult. The intense hunger will cause you to binge eat, or to feast whenever you break your fast. Consuming the additional calories will then cause you to gain weight as opposed to losing it.

The low-carb ketogenic diet also results in mental sharpness and acuity. There is plenty of scientific evidence that seems to suggest that ketones improve our cognitive abilities and mental functioning. The western diet, which typically consists of foods that are rich in refined carbohydrates, has been proven to result in the degradation of the nervous system, resulting in reduced memory and cognitive abilities.

In addition, ketones are believed to boost mental abilities since they are a much more efficient source of energy. Fats are more powerful because they contain much more energy for every unit of oxygen that is utilized. Glucose is used up more quickly compared to fats. As such, fat is a more constant source of energy for the brain.

Intermittent fasting is also beneficial to the ketogenic diet. The cycles of the eating and fasting windows ensure that the insulin levels in the bloodstream are low, resulting in higher ketone levels in the bloodstream. Higher ketone levels convert the body into a fat-burning machine resulting in weight loss.

Furthermore, intermittent fasting works through calorie restriction. The methods of intermittent fasting ensure that your daily calorie intake is significantly less than what a normal person on a three-meal-a-day approach is consuming because of the restricted feeding window. Better still, some methods of intermittent fasting ensure that your calorie intake is low whether you are feeding on healthy and nutritious meals, or unhealthy meals. Hence, intermittent fasting allows you to restrict your calorie intake while on the ketogenic diet.

Intermittent fasting also leads to the production of a protein called brain-derived neurotrophic factor (BDNF) within the nerve cells. The protein leads to improved learning, memory, and increases the production of new nerve cells. Animal studies have found that it also makes brain neurons resistant to dysfunction and degeneration.

12.3 How to Maximize the Benefits of Both Intermittent Fasting and the Ketogenic Diet

There are many benefits that you will expect to enjoy when you combine the ketogenic diet with intermittent fasting. They include: reduced hunger and cravings, increased energy levels, reduced moodiness and crankiness, improved mental functionality, increased insulin sensitivity, lower blood sugar, and efficient weight loss.

To enjoy these benefits, you will need to put in place some steps and measures that will ensure that you maximize these benefits. They are listed below:

1. Consult your medical practitioner before you start. This is especially the case if you suffer from any known medical conditions, such as diabetes and high blood pressure, if you are pregnant, or if you are breastfeeding.
2. Set your goals: You will need to analyze your eating habits, current weight, and any health conditions that you may have. Then create a game plan that involves the combination of the ketogenic diet and intermittent fasting, which will lead you to your goal. Inasmuch as losing weight is the ultimate goal, individuals should create smaller milestones to motivate them to move closer to the goal.
3. Surround yourself with positive energy: Avoid keeping the company of people who persistently remind you of your weight. Instead, surround yourself with people who are positive, and encourage you to become your best self. For added motivation, you could join a slimming club, which is a great way to meet new people who share the same goals as you.

4. Make sure your goals are realistic and attainable: Remember that the journey of a thousand miles starts with a single step. It doesn't matter how small you start, just as long as you start. This will provide you with a platform to work towards your ultimate goal.
5. Keep track of all your activities: You could track yourself using a food diary, an exercise log, or a spreadsheet that contains both records. By keeping track of your fitness exercises, eating habits, and even your moods, you become more accountable to yourself, and are motivated to achieve your next goal.
6. The ketogenic diet primarily involves the consumption of meals that contain high amounts of fats and oils, moderate amounts of protein, and low amounts of carbohydrates. Generally, the meals should also minimize the total calories which are being consumed. To maximize the weight loss process, you must ensure that all ingredients that you select meet the above

criteria. This will reduce the glucose levels in the bloodstream, and consequently, the levels of insulin. As such, the body will turn to its fat reserves as a source of fuel. The burning of fats will then result in weight loss.

7. The amount of carbohydrates that you consume should be minimized as much as possible. This is because feeding on high-carb foods while fasting intermittently will cause your blood sugar levels to rise whenever you break your fast, and to drop significantly during your fasting window. Unstable blood sugar levels will negatively impact the intermittent fasting process, as they will result in sleepiness, low energy, mood swings, and intense cravings.

8. Ketosis is a process that allows the body to burn down its fat reserves as a source of energy and fuel. When high-carb foods are broken down, glucose is released into the bloodstream and the body reverts to its natural state of breaking down glucose for energy. As such, you should avoid high-carb foods because they terminate the process of

ketosis and could result in weight gain, which goes against your main objective for intermittent fasting.

9. High fats and oils in the ketogenic diet are important to the intermittent fasting process because they provide the muscles and body organs with all the important minerals and nutrients that are required. In addition, fats and oils keep you satiated, reducing the occurrence of hunger pangs and cravings, which greatly impacts an individual's ability to fast for long periods of time. Fats and oils also result in improved mental performance and a reduction in inflammation.

10. While the ketogenic diet allows for foods that contain high fats, moderate proteins, and low carbohydrates, you should always abstain from eating unhealthy fats and proteins. Saturated fats have the potential of increasing your cholesterol levels. This is harmful to your health and could result in cardiovascular disease and other heart diseases. You should therefore avoid eating the following foods: fatty cuts of beef and

pork, foods that have been deep fried, some dairy products such as cream, cheese, and butter.

11. The ketogenic diet should therefore be well balanced and should largely contain unprocessed foods. Some of the foods that are recommended include: lean cuts of beef, pork, lamb and goat meat, fish, nuts, olive oils, seeds, whole grains, fruits, and vegetables. Such a diet is extremely nutritious and is likely to result in the longevity of your life, improved immunity, and reduced constipation.

12. Calorie-free beverages are also very important as they provide you with the desired hydration to keep your body in perfect shape. Coffee is particularly considered to be very important as it increases the metabolism of the body, leading to the increased burning of fat as a source of energy. In addition, coffee is important in reducing hunger pangs and cravings.

13. Identify the days of the week and schedule specific periods in the course of the day or the week in which you will have your meals, or those in which you will fast. The timings can always be changed depending on your schedule and bodily needs.
14. Repeat the process. As mentioned earlier, the ketogenic diet and intermittent fasting are a way of life, and you cannot expect the results to be visible within one day, one week, or even one month. The intended results will come as a result of consistency and dedication in the pursuit of your goal.
15. The first meal of the day, which is meant to break the fast, should be modest in size. Breaking the fast with a very large meal, or through binge eating, will slow down the fat burning process in your body making you tired. As such, the first meal that you consume after breaking your fast should contain 300 – 500 calories.

Your Quick Start Action Step:

Schedule some time to carry out in depth research and to consult a medical practitioner to provide you with all the knowledge that you will need before starting the ketogenic diet and intermittent fasting. This is especially so if you are suffering from any known medical conditions such as diabetes and high blood pressure, if you are pregnant, or breastfeeding.

Armed with the necessary knowledge, you could follow the steps highlighted above to schedule your fasting and feeding window, to create a suitable meal plan and to plan any workouts that you plan to engage in.

To create a comprehensive and conclusive meal plan, you will need to go out and shop for some of these foods and ingredients to restock your refrigerator and kitchen cabinets.

As you pursue this journey, you will need to realize that it is not for everyone. It will test your will and determination countless times. Hence, you will need to constantly motivate yourself and keep the company of positive people, preferably people who are pursuing the same goal. You could also frequently track your progress by recording it in a spreadsheet.

If you do not meet your goals, do not be hard on yourself. You will need to realize that fasting is difficult and find ways to motivate yourself to get back on track.

If you feel weak, dizzy, sluggish, moody, constantly tired, or experience some brain fog, you may need to stop the ketogenic diet and intermittent fasting process and seek the advice of your medical practitioner. You will need to realize that all human beings are fundamentally different and run your own race. After all, life is not a competition.

Bonus Book Preview: 'Keto Diet for Beginners: Your Ultimate & Essential Step-by-Step Ketogenic Lifestyle Guide to Losing Weight Fast and Eating Better for Long-Term Weight Loss, Healthy Living and Feeling Good' by Amy Maria Adams

Chapter 1: Getting Started with the Keto Diet for Beginners

1.1 Definition of the Keto Diet

The ketogenic diet, also called the keto diet for short, is simply a diet that is high in fat and low in carbohydrates. It is also sometimes called low-carb, high-fat diet, or simply low-fat diet. The diet aims at reducing the intake of carbohydrates and replacing them with fat; this has many health advantages. By reducing the consumption of carbohydrates, the body is put in a metabolic state known as ketosis which is an increase in the number of ketone bodies in the blood.

When on a ketogenic diet, the body initiates a natural phenomenon in order to help us survive whenever food intake is low; this leads to efficiency in the way the body burns fat for energy. Also, fat is turned into ketones in the liver, which supplies energy for the brain; this is because the body is naturally adaptive to whatever is put into it. When there's an overload of fats and a reduction of carbohydrate intake, the body then begins to rely on ketones as its primary source of energy.

When not on a keto diet, the body relies on glucose as its source of energy, and therefore, fats are stored since they are not needed. The body chooses glucose over any other energy source because it is easy to convert. However, while on a keto diet, the body is deprived of that needed glucose, thereby forcing the body to depend on other sources of energy, in this case, fats. The ketogenic diet has recently become popular for weight loss amongst celebrities.

Who invented the keto diet?

Over the years, various dietary cures have been suggested for curing epilepsy, and many such treatments had to do with the increase or reduction of many substances like animals, vegetables, or minerals. Also, even though medical practitioners have adopted fasting as a mode of treatment for many sicknesses and ailments for more than two and a half thousand years now, fasting as a cure for seizures is not officially recognized.

The Hippocratic collection of the 5th Century BC recorded fasting as its sole treatment for epilepsy. During the fifth century BC, Hippocrates wrote about a man who had an epileptic attack. Total abstinence from food and drink was the cure for the attack.

By the early twentieth century, the ketogenic diet had been used medically as a way of replicating the biochemical impacts that a fast (or starvation) would have. The earliest scientific reports that exist about the importance of fasting in epilepsy were written by French physicians Guillaume Guelpa and Auguste Marie.

It was Dr. Russell M. Wilder, an American doctor at the Mayo Clinic, that coined the term ketogenic diet.

Dr. Wilder suggested, most likely based on the work written by Woodyatt who was also a renown medical expert, "that the advantages of fasting could be acquired if ketonemia was supplied to the body by a different means. The ketone bodies are made from fat and protein at whatever point an imbalance exists between the measures of fatty acid and sugar that are consumed in the tissues. Regardless, as has for quite some time been known, it is possible to incite ketogenesis by encouraging diets which are exceptionally rich in fat and low in carbohydrates. It is proposed in this manner, to attempt the impacts of such ketogenic diets on a set of people with epilepsy." Wilder suggested that a ketogenic diet is as effective as fasting and can be sustained for a more extended period, thereby compensating for the obvious detriments of a prolonged fast.

In a report issued the next day, he depicted the surprising improvement in the seizure control of three of his epileptic patients who were admitted to the Mayo Center to be put on the ketogenic diet. He stated that, "It is difficult to reach conclusions from the results of these set of patients who were treated with high-fat diets, yet we have here a strategy for watching the impact of ketosis on the person with epilepsy. If this is the instrument responsible for the significant impact of fasting, it might be possible to substitute for that somewhat harsh method of dietary treatment which the patient can pursue with a lesser level of inconvenience and continue at their homes as long as it seems necessary."

How the ketogenic diet works

The primary source of ketone bodies for the body is via ketogenesis. The raw materials used for this process are fatty acids in adipose tissues and amino acids that are ketogenic. Adipose tissues usually serve as a site for fat storage, and this helps in the regulation of body temperature and as an energy reserve. These stored up fatty acids can be released by a hormone known as an adipokine, which is any of the several cytokines secreted by the adipose tissue, signaling that the body has a high level of glucagon and epinephrine, and hence a low insulin level. This state connotes periods of starvation or when the glucose level in the blood is low. For the metabolism of fatty acid to lead to energy production, it must occur within the mitochondria. However, free fatty acids cannot successfully transport through the biological membrane without help; this is due to the negative electric charge they carry.

As crazy as it sounds, the way the ketogenic diet works is that to lose fat, you have eat fat; this is possible because the body is put in a state of full reliance on fats where instead of storing fats, it burns fats for energy. The body is naturally programmed to run on glucose, but while on the keto diet, carbohydrate intake is very low and therefore means little glucose will be available for the body to use. Hence, the body then changes its source of energy from glucose to ketones from fats. The body becomes a fat burning machine.

What does the ketogenic diet consist of?

A ketogenic diet is a diet that contains very low carbs and very high-fat content. It shares a lot of similarities with low-carb diets and the Atkins diet. In a keto diet, fat intake is primarily replaced with carbohydrate consumption. The aim is to obtain more calories of your daily meal from protein and fat rather than from carbs.

The drastic reduction in the intake of carbohydrates makes your body begin to adapt to such changes, therefore putting your body in a metabolic state known as ketosis. When this occurs, your body becomes an efficient "fat-burning machine." Due to a massive reduction in sugar intake, the body responds to this by converting fat into ketones, to serve as an alternative source of energy for the brain, since the brain cannot utilize fat.

Who benefits from ketogenic diets?

Being on a keto diet has numerous benefits ranging from weight loss, to reduced hunger, to improved memory retention. A ketogenic diet can help in improving health conditions such as diabetes and cardiovascular disease. Usually, any diet that aids in the excessive burning of body fat and weight reduction can reduce the risk of diabetes and certain cardiovascular diseases. And, in general, any diet that helps reduce and stabilize blood glucose, keeps blood pressure in check, and reduces triglyceride levels can prevent heart disease.

What is ketosis?

Ketosis is a state in the body in which ketone bodies in the blood are used as a primary energy source, as opposed to the state in which the glucose contained in the blood serves as the primary energy source. Usually, ketosis is said to occur when the body utilizes fat at a rapid rate, leading to the conversion of fatty acids to ketones. The state of ketosis means that the body has switched from depending on carbohydrates to burning fat for fuel. As a person lessens his or her carbohydrate intake and increases dietary fats, more fat is metabolized, and ketone bodies are created. Most fats are essential to the body and do not affect heart disease risk. Fatty acids (fat) and amino acids (protein) are necessary for living. The keto diet is a low carbohydrate, high-fat diet. A standard diet is about 50 percent carbohydrates, 35 percent fat, and 15 percent protein, but the keto diet is about 70-75 percent fat, 15-20 percent protein, and about 10 percent carbohydrates. A ketogenic diet reduces the risk factor for heart diseases like stroke, epilepsy, etc. In ketosis, your body is using ketone energy for strength instead of glucose. Entering ketosis can take a little more than three days once a person begins the keto diet. At that point, a person is using fat for energy instead of carbohydrates. The keto diet promotes fresh food like meat, fish, vegetables, and healthy fat and oils. The calorie is an essential factor in the formation of ketones. A calorie is a unit of energy. Calorie consumption dictates weight gain or loss. The macronutrient is another factor in the creation of ketones. Macronutrients are found in all foods and are measured in grams (g) on nutrition labels. Fat contains nine calories per gram while protein contains four calories per gram and carbohydrates provide four calories per gram. On a keto diet, 70-75 percent of the calories one eats should come from fat.

Ketosis is a nutritional state in which the concentration of insulin (the hormone associated with fat storage) and blood glucose is at a shallow and stable level. It is associated highly with hyperketonemia, that is, an increased level of ketone bodies within the blood. Ketones, though they can be acquired through the consumption of ketone supplements, can also be produced within the body by a process known as ketogenesis in which the glycogen stored within the body is biochemically broken down. Long-term ketosis can be a result of abstaining from food or eating a low-carb diet (keto diet). Self-induced ketosis comes with medically related benefits, e.g., curing different types of diabetes, epileptic seizure reduction, appetite control, brain injury protection, athletic performance, etc.

When glucose (glycolysis) is used as the primary source of energy, insulin levels are usually at a high level, promoting fat storage, while, in ketosis, stored-up fat is typically utilized. Because of this, ketosis is sometimes called the "fat- consuming" state.

The primary ketone bodies used as an energy source are acetoacetate and beta-hydroxybutyrate. The two hormones majorly responsible for the concentration of ketone bodies in the body are glucagon and insulin. In a normal state, most cells make use of both glucose and ketone bodies for energy.

It is important to know that ketosis is entirely different from ketoacidosis, the significant difference being in the ketone levels present in the blood. Whereas ketosis is the adapting of the body to a low-carb environment, ketoacidosis, on the other hand, is life-threatening due to the alarming concentration of glucose and ketone bodies in the blood.

Abstaining from carbohydrates to the extent of ketosis is said to have both pros and cons on a person's health. Ketosis can be stimulated by periods of starvation, or after the consumption of ketone foods and supplement.

Diagnosis of ketosis

Ketosis can be detected using a specific urine test strip, for example, Ketostix and chemstrip kits.

• Ketostix are reliable for urine testing. The chemstrip is good for at least six months.

• Chemstrip kits are the second method that can be used to check urine ketones.

How to use the Ketostix

- Collect a fresh urine sample in a dry and clean container (mix the urine specimen properly before testing.)
- Perform the test in a well-lit area (any high moisture from the air will cause the strip not to work correctly.)
- Check the expiration date on the bottle of Ketostix. A new container of Ketostix can be used for six months after the first use. Always write down the day you first open the bottle on the bottle label as using the strips beyond the expiration date may lead to poor results.
- Remove one strip from the bottle. Wipe the edges of the strip along the rim of the urine container to remove excess urine. Then turn the test strip on its side and tap it once on a piece of absorbent paper.
- Hold the strip in a vertical position and compare reagent areas to the corresponding color list on the bottle label at the specified time.
- Read your results in good light.

If your test results are inconsistent or questionable:

- Check to confirm that the bottle has not

expired yet as seen on the label.
- Reconfirm your result by using another Ketostix, preferably from the same container.
- Alternatively, you can also obtain a new bottle of strips and retest the specimen.

The closer the color is to deep purple, the more ketones are in your body. Note that the test will be difficult to interpret for anyone color-blind.

Severity of ketosis

The level of ketone bodies differs based on diet, genetic influence, exercise, metabolic adaptation, etc. Ketosis can be stimulated by staying on a ketogenic diet for more than three days; this is usually referred to as "nutritional ketosis."

It is important to note that urine measurements do not equal blood measurements, as urine concentrations are usually more hydrated and therefore lower. After staying on a ketogenic diet for a while, the concentration lost in the urine may be reduced while the metabolism still relies on ketone bodies in the blood as an energy supply. Blood tests for ketones are much more reliable; however, the test strips are costly.

Urine ketone testing is notoriously unreliable. Most urine strips only detect acetoacetate levels, while, in a severe case of ketosis, the predominant ketone body will be beta-hydroxybutyrate. At any blood level, ketones are excreted into the urine; this is quite the opposite when it comes to glucose. Ketoacidosis is a disorder that can't take place within a healthy individual who secretes insulin normally.

Controversies about ketosis

Some health experts consider abstinence from carbohydrate diets unhealthy. However, achieving a state of ketosis does not require the complete elimination of carbohydrates from the menu. Other health experts regard ketosis as a simple metabolic process that is characterized by fat-burning. Ketosis, which is usually followed by gluconeogenesis, is the particular state that worries some health experts. However, it is rare for a person in good health to reach a dangerous keto level. Individuals who suffer from the inability to secrete basal insulin are more likely to reach a life-threatening level of ketosis, eventually leading to a coma.

Signs and symptoms that can help you know if you are in ketosis

You can monitor your ketosis level using a urine or blood strip, but these are quite expensive. Alternatively, you can use specific "markers" to know if you've got it right:

- **Frequent urination** – The keto diet is a diuretic and therefore increases the rate of urine excretion. Acetoacetate, a ketone body, is usually excreted with urine.
- **Dry mouth** – the increased urination usually leads to an increase in thirst and a dry mouth. Hence, ensure you stay hydrated in order to regulate your electrolytes.
- **Mouth odor** – acetone is a ketone body that smells like an overripe fruit; it is released when we breathe. This odor gradually is reduced over the long-term.
- **Curbs hunger levels and increase energy** – a reduced hunger level usually characterizes the ketosis state.

Discomforts you may suffer during the first few weeks of being in ketosis

Your body is already well familiar with the

normal process of utilizing carbohydrates as an energy source. Over time, the body secretes myriad enzymes to assist this process, but only a few enzymes associated with the breaking down of fat.

And all of a sudden, your body has to adapt to the reduction in glucose level and increase in total fat intake, which means having to build up an entirely different arsenal of enzymes. As your body initiates a state of ketosis, your body will utilize its remaining glucose reserve, breaking down glycogen in the muscles, which can cause a reduction in performance and lack of energy.

During the first week, many individuals complain of dizziness, headaches, etc. This is usually the side effects of the loss of most of your electrolytes, as ketosis increases the rate of urine excretion. These can be countered by drinking plenty of water and increasing your salt intake.

Sodium will aid with water retention and assist in replenishing flushed-out electrolytes.

What is a macro? And how to measure it?

Macros, also known as macronutrients, are fats,

proteins, and carbohydrates. They play a vital role in providing our body with essential nutrients and acting as a primary energy source for our daily activities; this is what earns them the term "macro," meaning "large." We not only need them for the proper functioning of our body system, but we also need them to live.

Macro-measuring means to measure the macronutrients in your diet to ensure you're consuming the ideal daily amount of fats, proteins, and carbohydrates, although the perfect amount of each differs from individual to individual depending on certain factors like lifestyle, metabolism, and age. In other words, when measuring your macros, you will need to understand your body and what it needs. Knowing your body well may take a bit of time, but it's worth it.

- **Mesomorph** – this body type is naturally strong and muscular, with broad shoulders and very dense bones. Gaining or losing weight is moderately easy, while gaining muscle mass is very easy. Individuals in this category will require a macro constituent of 40-50 percent carbs, 35-45 percent protein, and 25-35 percent fat.

1.2 Benefits of keto diets

The ketogenic diet differs from other diets in the sense that many of those diets offer weight loss as their main advantage. The ketogenic diet comes with a large number of benefits because of the way it alters the chemical composition of the body. The keto diet leads to an increase in the production of ketones, as well as a dependence on ketones for the daily maintenance of the body. The body is more efficient when it depends on ketones as fuel. Amongst the many advantages of the ketogenic diet, a few will be discussed below:

- **Weight loss** – because of its low carbohydrate content, the ketogenic diet brings about a breaking down of body fat into ketones and allows the body to depend mainly on ketones rather than glucose. In other words, the fat stored up in the body will be used as a source of energy. When an individual is on a keto diet, insulin, which is the fat-storing hormone level, drops massively, turning the body into a fat-consuming machine since fat storage is prevented. Scientifically, on long-term analysis, a regularly practiced ketogenic diet has proven to show better results as compared to low-fat and high-carb diets; cholesterol is produced from the conversion of excess glucose in the diet. Ketogenic diets generally have an improved feeling of satiety, hence leading to an overall reduction in food intake. This allows for reduced calorie intake without necessarily causing ravenous hunger.

- **Increase in the levels of HDL cholesterol** – whenever people hear about an increase in the level of cholesterol, there is usually a panic, and this is because many are not well informed that there are two types of cholesterol (the HDL and the LDL). The HDL is the one that is more needed because it carries cholesterol from the body to the liver (the liver is where it can be reused or excreted.) Conversely, the LDL transports cholesterol from the liver to all parts of the body.

1.3

One of the ways you can find out how much you know, do not know or need to know about the keto diet as a beginner and is to take online tests. That's a good way of checking your knowledge base (if it's sound enough) and there are many websites where you can take such tests. You can take tests at "Completely Keto" at http://completelyketo.com or "Bhu Foods" at http://bhufoods.com

Your Quick Start Action Step:

Create some time before the end of the day to take the test at any of the websites listed above and take the tests.

None of the tests should take more than 15 to 20 minutes.

Chapter 2: The Ketogenic Diet – Common Questions Answered

2.1 Is the ketogenic diet safe?

It is normal that whenever a new diet hits the scene, there's always information that talks about its negative impacts on your health. However, what is the case with the keto diet? The keto diet has undergone scientific tests and analysis and has been recommended by great medical institutions globally. It has been proven to be safe; however, this depends on the activity level and condition of the individual. But on a general scale, it is entirely safe. It is helpful for achieving a healthy lifestyle and not just a miracle cure.

2.2 Does the ketogenic diet work?

The ketogenic diet has been in use for a very long time; it became more pronounced in the 1920s and since then has been used repeatedly on different individuals. The keto diet started as a cure for epileptic children, with many of them being completely cured. The ketogenic diet has been proven to work for many conditions starting from weight loss to heart disease. Its impact on weight loss has been debated as a short-term impact; some patients apparently regain weight after about a year or two. But this is highly debatable.

2.3 Does the ketogenic diet work for the long-term?

It is highly debatable whether the use of ketogenic diets for weight loss works for the long-term; however, it is not medically or scientifically proven otherwise. Using weight loss for other diseases works, for example, for people with diabetes, and the cure is long-term. The same thing applies to high-blood pressure if they are able to follow through with the diet successfully.

2.4 Does the ketogenic diet affect weight loss?

The answer is yes. The ketogenic diet is gaining popularity again not precisely because of its benefits for other diseases but because of its use for weight loss. The ketogenic diet is beneficial for weight loss because of the dramatic reduction in the intake of carbohydrates, forcing the body to burn fat as its source of energy rather than glucose from carbohydrates. It also reduces appetite, which also contributes to weight loss. By affecting appetite, it reduces individuals' cravings for sugar.

2.5 How does a ketogenic diet affect cholesterol?

It is a common misconception that since ketogenic diets are high in fat content, they lead to an increase in cholesterol levels in the body. However, this is not true. Much scientific research has shown that low-carb diets help in optimizing the cholesterol level in the body. Many are unaware that there is good cholesterol and bad cholesterol. HDL cholesterol is the one known as "the good cholesterol." It collects all cholesterol that is not in use within the body and takes it to the liver, where it is either recycled or destroyed. The ketogenic diet causes a reduction in LDL, "the bad cholesterol," which is responsible for some cardiovascular diseases in adults.

2.6 What is the "keto flu" and how do you minimize it?

Starting a keto diet can be very strange. You have a lot to look forward to including a lot of weight loss and a lot of anticipated internal changes that your body is bound to undergo. However, keto flu is something else that might also come along when starting a keto diet. Your body may experience keto flu during the initial stages of being on a keto diet. Usually, the body gets a little weak before it finally starts getting stronger. The extent to which your body suffers usually depends largely on your previous diet as it determines the shock your system will undergo from your new diet pattern; the effect of that shock is what you will begin to experience.

Once you start a keto diet, some symptoms are sure markers of having the keto flu. They include:

- Headaches

- A cough

- Fatigue

- Irritability

- Nausea

These symptoms are usually indications that your body needs to adjust to the changes in your diet pattern and adapt to what you're putting it through. Having these symptoms is not enjoyable, and it sucks; they can leave you discouraged and make you wonder whether it is worth the pain and discomfort. However, these symptoms will eventually fade away as your body approaches ketosis. These symptoms are just your body reacting to carb deprivation, but over time, these symptoms will go just as quickly as they came.

A ketogenic diet contains a very low-carb content, and therefore your body tries to adapt to the low intake of carbs since you have been consuming a large amount of carbs your whole life up to this point. Staying away from carbs will tend to come as a shock to your body, but very soon your body will recover and continues on the path to good health. When suffering from the keto flu, you may start to consider eating more carbs to make the pain and discomfort go away, but do not listen to this temptation; endure for a couple of days, and everything will go back to normal.

How to minimize the flu?

Once on a keto diet, one of the numerous changes your body will undergo is a loss of body fluids and electrolytes in the form of sodium, potassium, and magnesium. Electrolytes are vital to the proper functioning of your body as they play a significant role in determining the amount of water in your body and how effectively your muscles perform their task. Carbs usually help with water retention within the body, ensuring there is no excessive loss of electrolytes. When staying on a keto diet, you will begin to lose a lot of body fluids, and since most electrolytes are dissolved in these fluids as a solvent, it is natural that you will lose some of them. Also, since your body is going to be consuming a lot of stored-up body fat, and your body cells will begin to replace these fats with water, it is essential to stay hydrated. It is also necessary to add a lot of salt to your daily meal by eating foods that have a high sodium content. If your electrolyte consumption is high, then you'll be just fine.

How long will it take for my body to adjust?

When on a regular diet, your body is, necessarily, sugar dependent but when on a keto diet, your body becomes fat dependent. This kind of change usually has a drastic effect on the body, but time is all your body requires. The adjustment period differs with individuals. However, on average, it takes more than a week to finally reach the ketosis stage; for some, it occurs faster than that. It all depends on how your body reacts to the effect of such changes; this is the time your body begins to shed some fat. It is essential to note that even when your body has reached the ketosis stage, that doesn't mean it will stay in it when you begin to eat carbs again. Some individuals can get away with it; others can't. It is just safer to adhere strictly to your diet.

2.7 How many carbs can I eat on the keto diet?

The amount of carbs every individual needs is dependent on a couple of things. Generally, eating less carbs has more impact. It will speed weight loss and reduce appetite and hunger. Someone with type 2 diabetes should eat fewer carbohydrates; it will improve insulin resistance. The truth is that many people find a diet that is very low in carbs somewhat too challenging and restrictive.

2.8 How much protein should I eat on the keto diet?

When on a keto diet, it is essential to eat a lot of

protein. However, if you eat too much of it, this will lower your ketone levels; if you eat too little, it leads to you losing excess muscle. So you should be at the midpoint in that sense. For someone that is sedentary, that is, you do a whole lot of sitting during the day, you should eat around 0.6 grams and 0.8 grams of protein for every pound of lean body mass. If you are someone who has an active day, you should eat between 0.8 grams and one gram of protein for every pound of lean body mass. If you want to gain some muscle, you should eat about one gram and 1.2 grams of protein for every pound of lean body mass. You don't need more protein than that.

2.9 What ketogenic diet is best?

In selecting the best diet, there are some things to consider. If you're someone who rarely engages in highly intense exercise and wants to lose weight, you should stick to the standard keto diet. If you add more carbohydrates, you will only be slowing down your progress and prolong how long it takes to reach ketosis, unlike those who don't add carbs. For people who engage in intense exercise regularly, then the cyclical keto diet and the targeted keto diet might be right for you. If you're someone who has only started intense workouts regularly within the last year, you should try out the targeted keto diet and see if you notice a decrease in performance while you're on the standard keto diet. When it comes to figuring out the best type of keto diet for you, it is important that you experiment. There are no individuals that are the same; you must find out what works for you best. It is important also to note that if you're not doing intense exercise regularly, then you should stay on the standard keto diet. Usually, most people do not need anything more than the standard keto diet.

To learn more about this book and how it can help you achieve a healthier lifestyle, search the title "Keto Diet for Beginners: Your Ultimate & Essential Step-by-Step Ketogenic Lifestyle Guide to Losing

Weight Fast and Eating Better for Long-Term Weight Loss, Healthy Living and Feeling Good" by Amy Maria Adams at the online store.

Conclusion

Thank you again for owning this book!

I hope this book was able to help you to understand how intermittent fasting can be used to lose weight, and to live a healthier lifestyle. In addition, I hope that the bonus chapter was helpful in linking intermittent fasting to the ketogenic diet.

So far, I hope you have come to understand that intermittent fasting is not merely a diet, but a way of life that comes with numerous health benefits for you. It is also my hope that you have come to appreciate the benefits that come with the intermittent fasting diet and have come to terms with the fact that it is not as extreme as people make it sound. In addition to the known benefits, you must be aware that intermittent fasting is a new concept, and that there are many more benefits that are still being explored and studied by nutritionist and medical practitioners.

Inasmuch as intermittent fasting and the ketogenic diet are perfect compliments in the weight loss journey, do not feel pressured to adopt both the methods since they still work perfectly when used independently. It is advisable that you begin with the ketogenic diet, then gradually incorporate the intermittent fasting method once you believe in yourself.

If you have started intermittent fasting and it feels uncomfortable at first, I would advise you to give yourself time to adjust. There is no standard duration of time that it will take you to adjust to fasting, as we are all inherently different and unique. Hence, simply monitor your body and understand some of the signals that it will be communicating to you.

Throughout the whole process, you must bear in mind that intermittent fasting will indeed test your discipline and willpower in ways that you cannot imagine or believe to be possible. However, here's a piece of encouragement; the beginning is the hardest part, it gets better! All you will need to do is to maintain a positive mindset and surround yourself with positive people, preferably those who share the same goals as you. In no time at all, you will find yourself able to fast for longer without experiencing any feelings of hunger or cravings.

To keep yourself motivated, you could maintain a record of your feeding habits and physical activities in a spreadsheet to help you monitor your progress, and to establish any trends that could provide opportunities for growth.

It cannot be stressed enough that intermittent fasting is not for everyone! As such, as soon as you begin the fasting process, you will need to carefully monitor your body for any signs of weakness, dizziness, light-headedness, moodiness, or even constipation. If you observe these symptoms, you are advised to stop the fasting diet and consult the experts moving forward.

Beginners should focus on having shorter fasting windows, and gradually work towards increasing the hours, as they gain more resilience and endurance. If you are unable to complete the fasting window without eating, do not be hard on yourself. Instead, take time to re-strategize to ensure that you do not fall again. To avoid breaking your fast prematurely, you could put in place gifting mechanisms where you will reward yourself for successfully completing the fasting window.

Anyone suffering from a health condition should be careful and consult the advice of a medical practitioner before starting the intermittent fasting diet. This is especially the case for people suffering from diabetes or high blood pressure. Such people should persistently monitor their blood sugar levels and blood pressure at least four times daily.

The next step is to implement everything that you have learned from this book. Feel free to make any amendments and modifications to suit you and your lifestyle. After all, you must always remember that the intermittent fasting diet is meant to fit into your life and not the other way around.

Bearing in mind that knowledge is power, you

should never stop reading, researching, or consulting on the intermittent fasting diet. Feel free to get the opinions of other people and frequently compare notes with them to stay motivated and optimistic. As such, now that you have successfully completed this book, start researching on the next book that you will be picking up.

Once you have gotten comfortable with intermittent fasting, you could slowly begin to incorporate a workout or fitness program to keep yourself physically fit. Due to the intensity of the program, you will need to only consider activities that are either light or moderate. To get the most out of your fitness program, you could consult a fitness expert who will create a workout plan for you.

In conclusion, you should always bear in mind that you are a social creature, and like all social creatures, you have social needs and demands. Hence, do not avoid going to celebrations or feasts because you are fasting. Occasionally give yourself a break and join other people to make merry. Later, you could compensate for this by fasting for extended periods of time or restructuring your feeding and fasting windows.

Thank you and good luck!

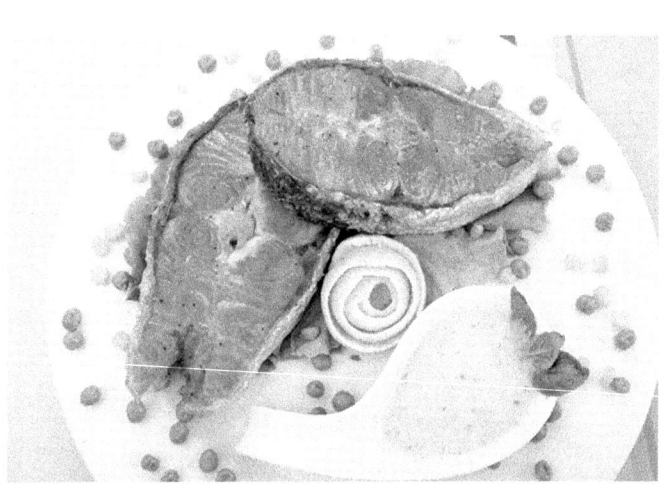

www.ingramcontent.com/pod-product-compliance
Lightning Source LLC
Chambersburg PA
CBHW051538020426
42333CB00016B/1993